Aesthetic Design
for Ceramic Restorations

David Korson

Dental Technician
London, England

Clinical Chapter by

A. C. S. Druttman MSc. BChD.

Quintessence Publishing Co Ltd 1994
London, Berlin, Chicago, São Paulo, Tokyo, Moscow,
Praha and Warshawa

First published 1994 by
Quintessence Publishing Company Ltd
London, UK

British Library Cataloguing in Publication Data
Korson, David
  Aesthetic Design for Ceramic Restorations
  1. Prosthetic dentistry
  I. Title
  617.69

  ISBN 1-85097-034-3

Printed and bound by Toppan Printing Co Pte Ltd, Singapore

from typesetting by Alacrity Phototypesetters.
Banwell Castle, Weston-super-Mare, UK.

Printed in Singapore

Foreword

David Korson is to be congratulated on producing a second book on ceramics since the time and effort involved in producing colour photographs of international standard requires great dedication, particularly when, in his case he is also running a busy commercial dental laboratory. The fact that he is at the sharp end of clinical practice accounts for the precision and quality of his photography and reflects his dedication to producing ceramic restorations that stand with the best that can be seen on the international lecture circuit.

His first chapter on the characteristics of natural dentitions is a delight and he has produced some beautiful colour reproductions of sections of natural teeth that reinforce his detailed descriptions of dentitions from youth to old age. Further chapters then deal with his methods of communication between dentist and technician and how these procedures can be translated into the reality of a ceramic restoration that is undetectable from its human counterpart. The use of diagnostic wax techniques is well illustrated and can save the technician time and money in translating the patient's expectations into a restoration that avoids conflict between all members of the dental team. David is also correct in emphasising the importance of constructing custom-built shade guides, indeed if only this became standard practice in all laboratories it would raise the standard of laboratory work overnight. His advice on communication through colour photography should also be heeded and his methods of using these transparencies to create the correct enamel overlays and dentinal effects complements his previous writing on natural ceramics.

The use of opalescent porcelains is described in depth and manufacturers are now producing sub-wavelength alumina or similar crystalline dispersed frits that offer the technician the opportunity of reproducing human enamel, without using over elaborate techniques. Although the production of opalescent porcelains dates back to the 1960s, it is only now that interest has been re-awakened in producing them for hand-built ceramics in the dental laboratory. However, as *David Korson* shows, fine ceramics are not so much dependent on the porcelains used as to how the technician interprets his viewing of the tooth and the skill with which he places his porcelain to reproduce this interpretation. His chapter on advanced laboratory techniques answers many of these questions.

The chapter by *Anthony Druttman* illustrates the importance not only of the precise preparation of teeth but also of the placement of crown margins in relation to the gingival tissue. The use of soft tissue models markedly assists the technician in producing the correct physiological contour to his crowns and this is well illustrated in the text.

David Korson is amongst the select few of dental technicians who spend time recording their work for posterity, only in this way can progress be judged by the ceramists following in his footsteps.

Dr *John W. McLean* OBE FDS RCS(Eng) MDS DSc(London) Dr Odont(Lund) DSc(LSU) President, International Society for Dental Ceramics. Consulting Professor in Fixed Prosthodontics and Biomaterials, Louisiana State University

Preface

The success of aesthetic and technical results place a heavy reliance upon the expertize of the dental technician. His place within the dental team is fundamental and, therefore, it is upon this that both dental surgeon and patient depend.

I firmly believe that to fulfil this duty technicians need to have direct access to the patient. To see first hand the oral situation and to have some involvement at the design stage of treatment planning.

Being involved in this way will provide valuable learning experience and the opportunity to assess results first hand will further improve the understanding of aesthetics.

Naturally this involvement must be limited to the aesthetic design of the restoration, discussion of the preparation and impression requirements and the indications for the various options of restorative materials.

It is in this way, with proper liaison between all partners in the 'team', that is, dentist, patient and technician, that a concerted effort for the benefit of the patient is assured.

David Korson

Acknowledgements

Preparing this volume has required considerable effort over a long period. The constant encouragement and support of my wife *Valerie* has helped me to accomplish this work. *Valerie* also prepared the illustrations and manuscript, for all of this my love and appreciation.

Sincere thanks to *Anthony Druttman* whose chapter on Tissue Management and Crown Contour added an extra dimension to the work. I am fortunate to know *Peter Gordon* whose advice on dental photography proved to be invaluable. Once again my thanks to Dr *John McLean* for reading the manuscript. A special thank you to Mr *H. W. Haase,* Mr *John Brooks* and the staff at Quintessence for their continued support and encouragement.

Contents

Contents

1 Studies of Natural Dentition

Today's aesthetic standards demand that artificial teeth are undetectable from their natural counterparts. Consequently, dental technicians need to gain first hand knowledge of natural tooth character and tooth structures to improve existing techniques.

For those who argue that their patients request white teeth, the sensible approach is to provide youthful teeth, which in reality is what the patient wants. Whether youthful or aged, all restorations need to be based upon nature's example through the study and simulation of the many characteristics of teeth, in this way more realistic ceramic restorations will result.

The purpose of this chapter is to highlight areas of tooth character which should enable both dentist and technician to simulate more natural restorations.

1.1 Characteristics of Natural Dentition

Physical Age of Dentition

Natural characteristics fall into groupings related to the age of the dentition, that is, young, middle-aged and aged. However, there is often a merging of age type. It is common to encounter a youthful dentition in a patient aged 40 years but equally, the aged characteristics of pits and crack lines are just as likely to be found in a patient of the same age. For this reason chronologic age is of less importance than the physiologic age of the dentition. Therefore, in the following descriptions of youthful, middle-aged and aged, it is the physiologic age of the dentition that is described.

Youthful dentition

The following examples illustrate typical characteristics common within this age group.

a) Blue/grey transparent incisal edge

b) Blue/grey proximal walls

c) Dentine colour halo effect surrounding incisal transparency (Rayleigh scattering)

d) Opalescent effects within the enamel layer

e) Dentine mamelons or random spots of dentine colour within the incisal region

f) White or off-white enamel faults or cracks

g) Enamel zones

h) Horizontal banding

i) Well defined Perikymata

j) Hypoplastic spots and patches

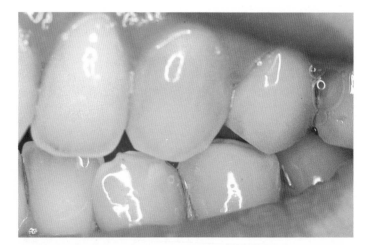

Figs 1 to 3 Typical of the young dentition, these examples exhibit a marked blue rim surrounding an inner dentine core. The incisal edge displays a pale dentine coloured halo effect. This is caused by light waves entering translucent enamel and being scattered by hydroxyapatite crystals within the enamel structure which are smaller than the wave length of light, termed Rayleigh scattering.

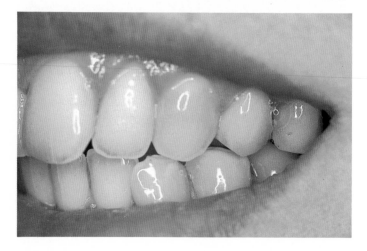

Fig 2

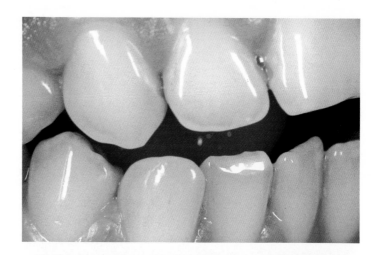

Fig 3

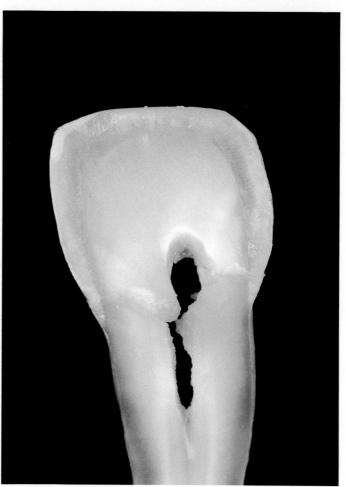

Fig 4 The mesiodistal longitudinal ground section clearly
shows the inner dentine core
and surrounding enamel.

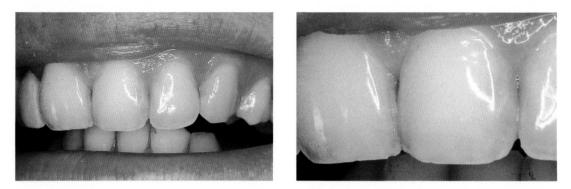

Figs 5 and 6 This mamelon structure is common to young dentition. These teeth are characterized by blue marginal ridges and three areas of mamelon colour.

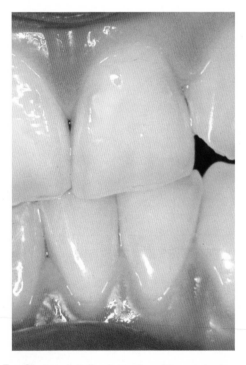

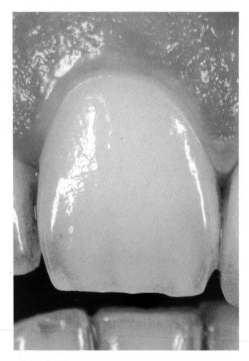

Fig 7 Close detail of teeth with mamelon structure extending to the incisal edge. Often, technicians assume the mamelon is a definite lobe formation within the tooth structure extending to within 1mm of the incisal edge, this is not always the case as can be seen by this example.

Fig 8 This patient, aged 35 years, has retained the blue proximal walls and dentine lobes, although the incisal edge has suffered some abrasion. This is an example of the merging of classic age band characteristics.

Middle-aged dentition

Characteristics for the middle-aged often overlap with both youthful and aged dentition. One cannot make assumptions that the typical characteristics for youthful dentition will not also be present in the middle-aged. The following list should be added to the list for the youthful dentition, to compile the many characteristics for the middle-aged.

a) Exposed root area
b) Discoloured crack lines
c) Discoloured spots or pits
d) Wear facets
e) Abrasion characteristics
f) Texture becoming smooth with satin-like surface lustre

Examples of middle-aged dentition

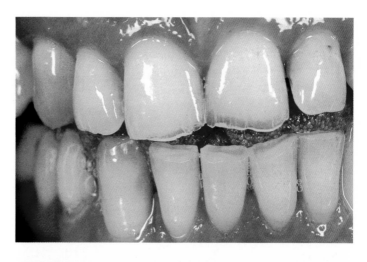

Fig 9 Representative of attrition at the incisal edges, these finely chiselled teeth display almost transparent enamel edges generating the white halo phenomena of Rayleigh scattering of light.

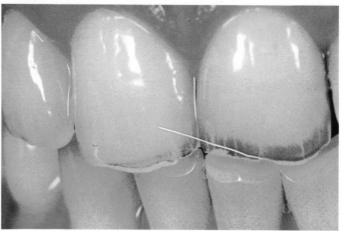

Fig 10 Close detail reveals the fine lamellae.

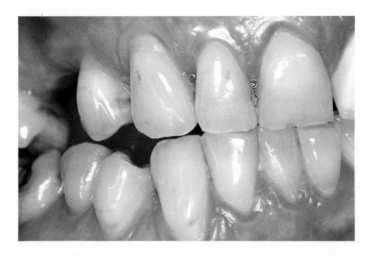

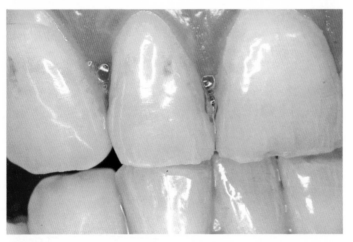

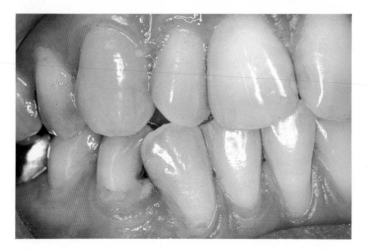

Figs 11 and 12 Middle-aged dentition with many distinguishing features

a) The incisal third displays slight brown discolouration beneath the enamel layer.
b) Faint enamel cracks, both white and discoloured.
c) Blue/grey tint at the proximal wall.
d) Faint blue/grey tint seen as a horizontal banding at the middle third of the facial aspect of the central incisor.
e) Dentine influence at the cervical third.
f) Surface staining.
g) Chipped incisal edges of central and lateral incisors.
h) Canine cusp displays wear facet.
i) Variations in shades between each tooth, canine is naturally the darkest.
j) Gingival recession has occurred on the canine and an area of exposed root surface is evident. Other teeth are beginning to display similar characteristics.
k) Polished smooth satin-like surface of the enamel.
l) Mandibular teeth display marked blue halo surrounding the dentine structure. The teeth are further characterized with surface staining of the interproximal areas and some labial surface spots.

Fig 13 Another example of middle-aged dentition. These teeth are characterized by the light enamel overlay of the central and lateral teeth contrasting with the dark colour of the canine.

Mandibular first bicuspid and canine teeth both exhibit gingival recession and root staining, typical characteristics in the middle and aged groupings.

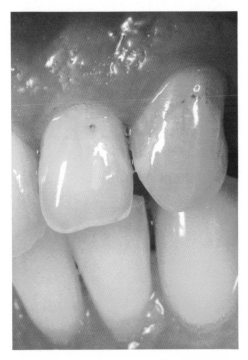

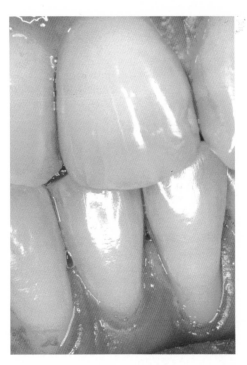

Fig 14 Lateral incisor is a classic example of middle-aged dentition. The translucency in the incisal third is clearly seen, surrounded by a dentine coloured halo. Discoloured pitting is evident around the course of the original tissue line.

Fig 15 Close detail of the central incisor discloses incisal characteristics of enamel lamellae and faint blue proximal margins.

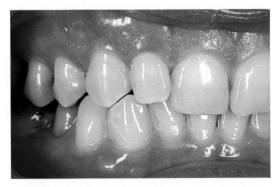

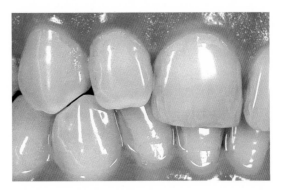

Fig 16 Many characteristics may be observed in this dentition. Once more the central incisor exhibits orange/brown discolouration within the incisal third, blue/grey proximal margins and some faint enamel lamellae. Lateral and canine teeth display a grey band at the mid-incisal third and a milky white incisal 1mm. Tooth surfaces are worn very smooth.

Fig 17 Close detail.

Aged dentition

The aged dentition is often typified by a thin layer of translucent enamel which allows dentine colours to show through clearly. Teeth appear smooth, with root areas often visible due to gingival recession and maxillary incisal edges worn flat. The mandibular incisal edge often display typical wear facets with exposed discoloured dentine and surrounding enamel rim.

Aged dentition requires similar characteristics to those aforementioned, however, the colouration becomes more intense and a further breakdown of enamel occurs. This is evident by the observation of:

a) Chipped incisal edges
b) Enamel pits and lesions
c) Discoloured composite resin restorations
d) Smooth surface texture and a high lustre

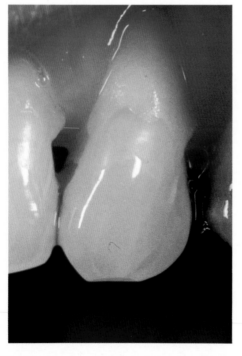

Fig 18   Highly translucent enamel with a blue hue and smooth glass-like appearance, typifying the aged dentition.

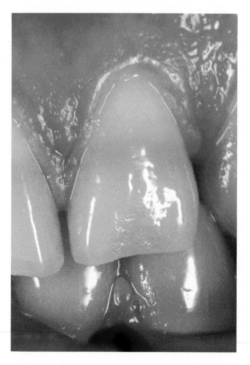

Fig 21   Close detail of the lateral incisor.

Fig 19 Translucent enamel allowing strong yellow/orange discolouration in the incisal area to filter through. Mandibular teeth appear to be losing chroma, mandibular lateral teeth are unworn and retain a blue enamel halo whilst the central incisors have been abraded and exhibit orange staining through the ingress of oral fluids.

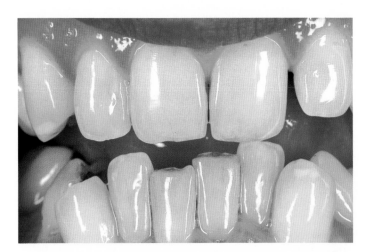

Fig 20 These teeth are characterized by the very obvious band of colour. In addition, yellow discolouration is evident in the incisal area of the lateral, the very different degrees of surface lustre between central and lateral teeth may be observed If lustre is low then low translucency occurs as a consequence.

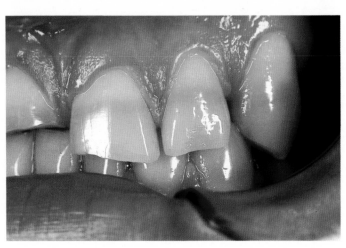

Enamel Cracks

Enamel cracks are common. In the young dentition they are only visible when viewed at an angle and would not be visible at all if it were not for the interruption of the light beam as it travels through the tooth surface. As the aging process occurs the crack gradually widens allowing the ingress of oral fluids, causing the crack to become stained.

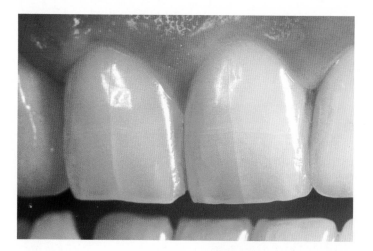

Fig 22 Enamel cracks in the young dentition.

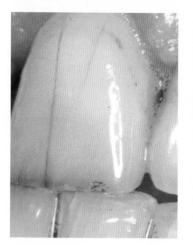

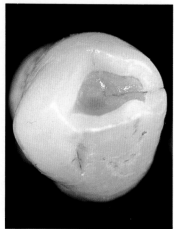

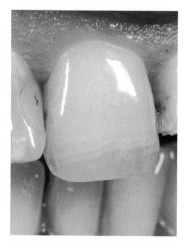

Fig 23 As the dentition ages the enamel crack becomes stained.

Fig 24 With the passage of time tooth abrasion has its effects, the mandibular incisors and canines are often severely attrited. This extracted tooth exhibits the archetypical incisal abrasion.

Fig 25 Horizontal lines occur frequently in all ages. In this example banding occurs in the body and incisal third of the tooth.

1.2 Ground Tooth Sections

Observation through tooth sections provides an invaluable insight in our search for information about the structure of teeth. With this technique enamel, dentine and pulp are all exposed to view, their stratification a source of enlightenment. Areas of opacity and transparency or translucency are easily observed, whilst even through low power magnification the enamel rods are clearly visible.

These and many other distinctive anatomical features will aid technicians in their endeavour to replicate natural dentition. Useful criteria may be utilized in discovering new ways to build layers of ceramic.

The Study of Tooth Structures

Tooth structure is composed of enamel, dentine and pulp, with a fine layer of cementum encompassing the root. Enamel, dentine and cementum are calcified tissue, surrounding the connective tissue of the pulp.

Physical proportions and composition

Enamel is semi-translucent and displays opalescent qualities. It is composed almost entirely of an inorganic material in the form of 89% Calcium Hydroxyapatite Crystals, 9% water and the remaining 2% organic material, by volume. The basic structure is rod or prism formation.

Dentine imparts the colour of tooth structure and is composed of 45% Calcium Hydroxyapatite Crystals, 30% organic material consisting of three connective tissue types: 1. odontoblasts (cells) 2. collagen (fibrous matrix) and 3. crown substance (carbohydrate molecules) and 25% water, by volume.

Dentine may be sub-divided into dentine and secondary dentine. Secondary dentine may be further divided into regular and irregular. Regular secondary dentine formation results through the ageing process and pathologic stimuli, as the pulp cavity decreases in size secondary dentine replaces it. Irregular secondary dentine is often caused through external stimuli such as attrition or caries, it is often observed filling the pulp form (fig 28).

Pulp is a connective tissue occupying the central area of the tooth from which root canals emanate, terminating in the apical foramen. The size of the pulp area decreases dramatically with age, preparation for crowning the tooth is severely limited until the late teen years. Composition of the pulp is 25% organic material and 75% water.

Cementum is a thin layer of calcified tissue encompassing the root portion

21

of the tooth, it varies in thickness from between 10μm to 600μm at the apex. Its function is to form part of the abutment between dentine and the periodontal ligament. Cementum is softer than dentine and is pale yellow in colour. (Berkovitz, Holland and Moxham, 1968. Renner, 1985)

Ground Sections Maxillary Central

(photographed with reflected light)

The dentine horn extends almost to the incisal edge. This is the cause of incisal characteristics, such as yellow influences.

Building dentine in a similar fashion prevents the incisal region appearing too grey, as in the typical body and tip

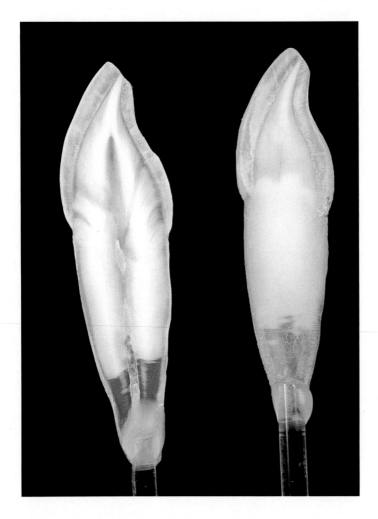

Fig 26 Longitudinal section through centre and distal portion. Enamel, dentine and pulp are clearly evident. Opacity is observed in the dentinal structure whilst a bluish translucency (opalescence) is seen in the enamel. The apical third of the root is almost transparent.

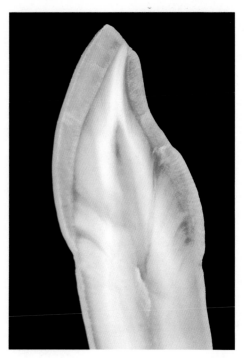 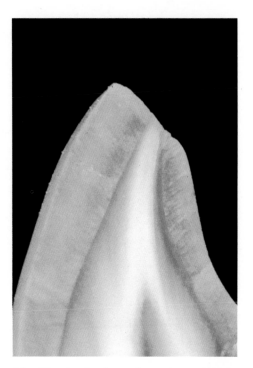

Fig 27 Coronal detail displays the amelodentinal junction mantle as an almost transparent line between dentine and enamel. The pulp is clearly observed as a thin clear/brown strip, whilst irregular secondary dentine formation continues to the incisal edge as an opaque white horn. Attrition has worn the enamel exposing the dentine.

Fig 28   Incisal section close detail
Stria of Retzius are clearly visible in the enamel band, especially at the palatal aspect. These are incremental lines running from the amelodentinal junction mantle to the surface. The stria are formed during the development of the enamel prisms and run obliquely across them. Details of the secondary dentine horn and amelodentinal junction mantle are also seen.

appearance of outmoded layering systems. Also note the morphology at the CEJ.

Stria of Retzius are evident on the tooth surface as a series of fine ridges known as perikymata. These vary from tooth to tooth and may become smooth, especially on the developmental ridges through wear and abrasion. Careful observance of these patterns will ensure realistic surface texture in ceramic restorations.

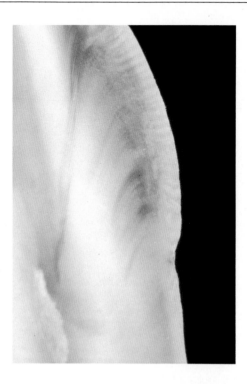

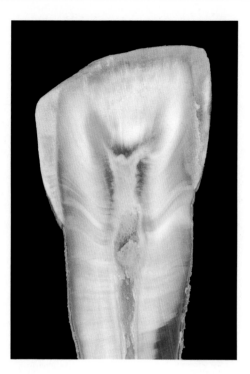

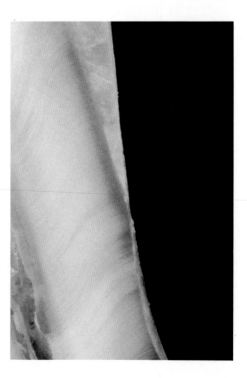

Fig 29   Cervical section close detail
Hunter-Schreger Bands within the enamel are observed within ground sections and are detected as light interacts with alternating directions of the enamel prisms.

Fig 30   Mesiodistal section
Anatomic structures observed from this view should be compared with fig 27.
   Dentine tubules are clearly seen. Note their course in different regions of the tooth.

Fig 31   Course of dentine tubules (section at the CEJ)
Close detail of the dentine tubules, the tubules taper from their pulpal end by 4μm to 1μm at the amelodentinal junction. (Berkovitz, Holland and Moxham, 1968) Observe the course of the tubules within the tooth structure.

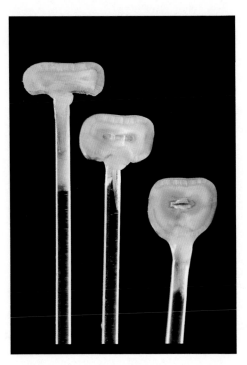

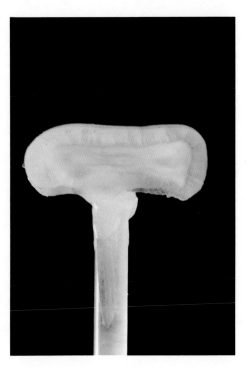

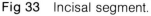

Fig 32   Horizontal sections (photographed with transillumination)
Incisal, body and cervical sections through the coronal part of a maxillary central display the various layers of tooth physiology quite dramatically. Variations in overall size of the structures are clearly seen.

Fig 33   Incisal segment.

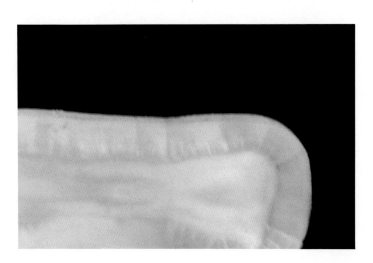

Fig 34   Incisal segment close detail. Note the enamel lamellae.

25

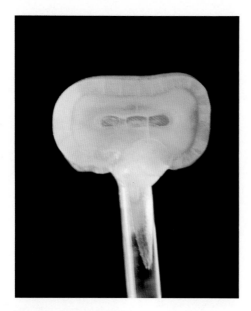

Fig 35 Body segment.

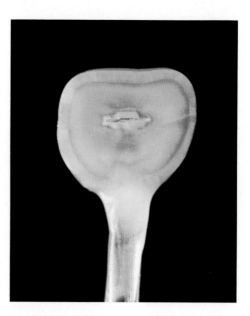

Fig 36 Cervical segment.

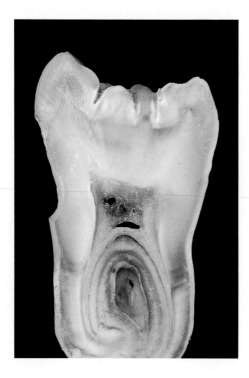

Mesiodistal sections of Mandibular Second Molar

Figs 37 to 39 Examples reveal enamel dentine and pulpal region in a facial plane. Enamel is noticeably thicker at the occlusal table, developmental fissures can be seen dividing the structure. Dentine horns are visible extending into the cuspal region. Pulpal region and root canal are clearly discernible.

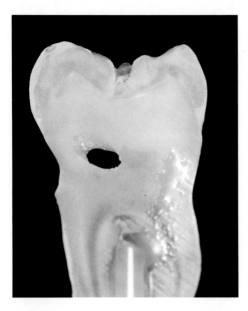

Fig 38

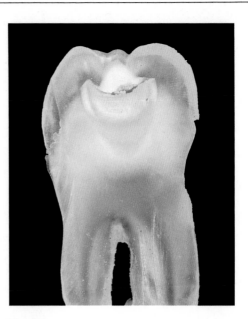

Fig 39

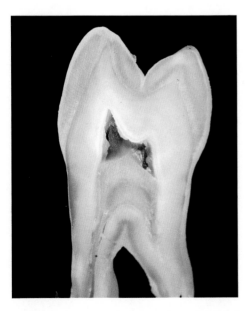

Fig 40 Reflected light. Longitudinal sections maxillary first molar.

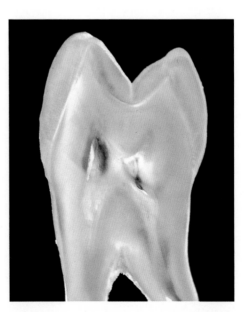

Fig 41 Transilluminated. Note the light reflection off the almost transparent amelodentinal junction mantle.

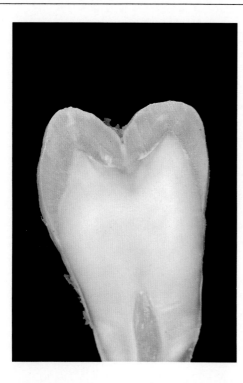

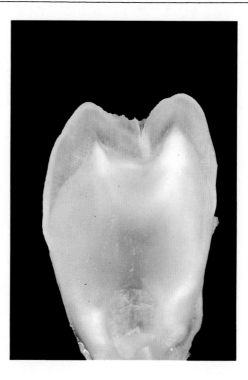

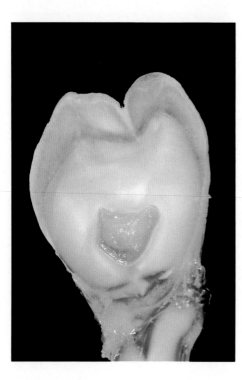

Figs 42 to 44 Mesiodistal sectons, mandibular first molar. Sections illustrate anatomic detail through the tooth segments.

Fig 42 Section through buccal cusps.

Fig 43 Section through central fossa.

Fig 44 Section through palatal cusp.

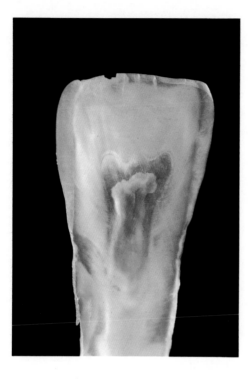

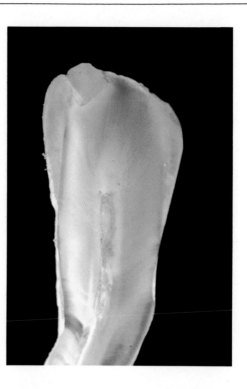

Tooth Sections Viewed Under Reflected Light and with Transillumination

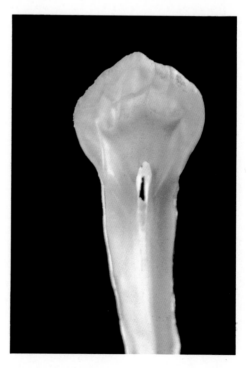

Figs 45 to 50 Mesiodistal sections demonstrate the anatomic details of the maxillary central, canine and bicuspid teeth in reflected light and with transillumination.

Note the orange/brown discoloration of the secondary dentine is due to abrasion of the cusp tip.

Figs 45 to 47 Transilluminated.

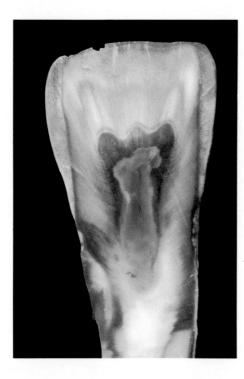

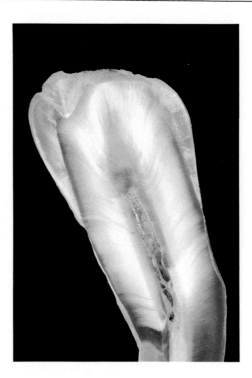

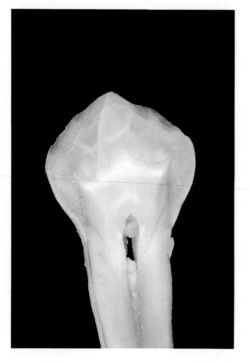

Figs 48 to 50 In reflected light.

Opalescence

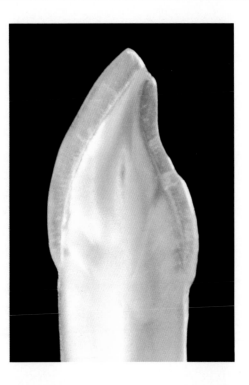

Figs 51 and 52 Photographed using a Philips 40 watt tungsten Reflecta bulb light source and Kodak EPY 64T tungsten film, these samples demonstrate the different spectral properties of tooth structure.

Fig 51 The light source is directed to provide reflected light.

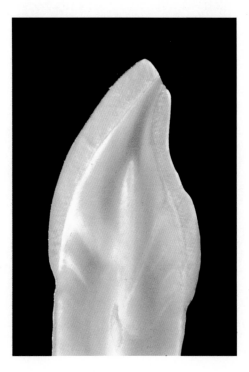

Fig 52 The light source is directed to provide transillumination.
  Tooth section displays opalescent properties as the light source is angled around the section.

Tooth Structures and their Relevance to Building Ceramics

Photographs of tooth sections make the structural anatomy quite clear, from which it can be seen that the enamel overlay covers the entire coronal portion of the tooth and this is the reason for depth of chroma and translucency. Therefore, in building ceramics it is important to bear this in mind and build a layer simulating enamel over almost the entire labial surface and much of the palatal surface.

New insight into the way light interacts with tooth tissue has brought further developments in ceramic engineering. These developments have led to improved ceramic materials which refract and absorb light in a way that is similar to that of natural dentition. (Yamamoto, 1989 and Sieber, 1993)

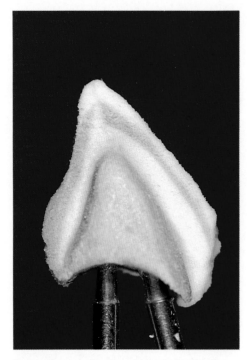

Fig 53 Vertical section through a typical ceramic build-up depicts porcelain layers which mimic natural dentition.

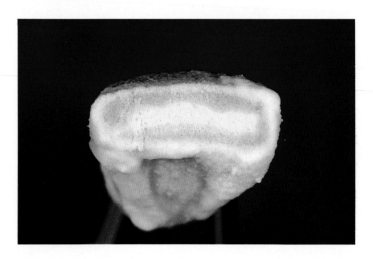

Fig 54 Horizontal section at the incisal third.

Further study of the photographs reveals secondary dentine development and its position within the structures and details of abrasion at the incisal edge. Regions of opacity and transparency are quite clearly evident.

References

1. *Berkovitz B. K., Holland G. R. & Moxham B. J:* A Colour Atlas and Textbook of Oral Anatomy. London. Wolfe Medical Publications Ltd. 1968.
2. *Renner R. P:* An Introduction to Dental Anatomy and Esthetics. Quintessence Pub. Co. Inc. Chicago. Illinois. 1985.
3. *Sieber C:* In the light of nature. QDT 16: 60 1993.
4. *Yamamoto M:* A newly developed 'Opal Ceramic' and its clinical use, with special attention to its relative refractive index. QDT 13. 1989.

2 Dentist — Technician — Patient Communication

Most would agree that close liaison between dentist and technician is essential if optimal results are to be achieved. It is a great shame that present protocol encourages only a summary meeting of the technician and patient to establish colours.

High standards in ceramics demand optimal involvement of the patient and a close working relationship between dentist and technician. Allowing the technician direct access to the patient provides greater opportunities for improved aesthetics.

This Chapter addresses in depth the way in which the dentist, technician and also the patient develop their relationships and the protocol which is necessary for further involvement between the patient and the technician.

2.1 Communication and Responsibility between Dentist and Technician

Communication is the key to success in this, as in all situations. The dentist-technician team have to prepare themselves to be in accord over procedural matters so that a cohesive team approach is presented. Meetings to discuss mutual concerns are beneficial. Shade control, preparation design and impression procedures are just a few areas where a close liaison is useful.

2.2 Patient Education by the Dentist

It is the dentist's responsibility to prepare the patient by explaining that to achieve the optimal restoration, the patient as well as dentist and technician must be disposed to make an effort. For the patient this means being prepared to spend as much time with the technician as is necessary, requiring high commitment and a great deal of understanding and patience.

The Communication Triad

The three partners in the team need to interact and each requires a clear understanding of the procedures that should be followed for a successful work pattern.

The following Table 1 is an example of a typical arrangement for the treatment of a patient requiring an aesthetic restoration.

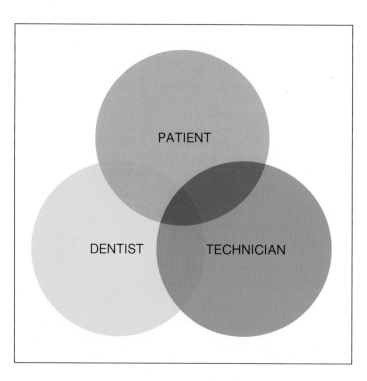

PATIENT

DENTIST   TECHNICIAN

Fig 55 The communication triad. A concept of the overlap for responsibility and involvement between patient, dentist and technician.

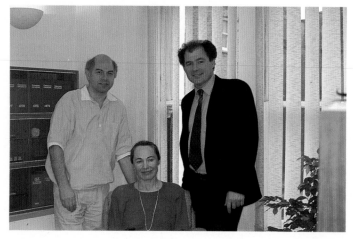

Fig 56 Anthony Druttman, with the patient and author, complete the triad necessary for optimal aesthetics.

Dentist — Patient	Dentist — Technician — Patient	Technician — Patient
1. Initiation for a particular form of treatment. The procedures, time frame, cost, advantages and disadvantages for all possible courses of treatment are explained. Alginate impressions for wax study.	2. Liaison between dentist and technician regarding technical details.	4. Patient visits the technician at the laboratory, where further detailed explanation of technical possibilities and initial shade selection takes place. In addition, a wax study* may be shown to the patient and alterations carried out in consultation with the patient.
	3. Meeting to discuss the possibilities for the suggested course of treatment and the opportunity for the dentist to introduce the patient to the technician.	
5. The teeth are prepared for the restorations and impressions taken. Final result of wax study is simulated in provisional restorations.		6. Aesthetic wax diagnostic trials have been fabricated and are tried in the mouth, alterations are carried out until satisfactory.
7. Restoration is tried in at the bisque stage, occlusion and marginal integrity are verified. Harmony with tissue contour is checked.		8. The bisque trial is tried in and alterations carried out to position and contour until the optimal result has been achieved. Stain, glaze and polish procedures are carried through and the bridge is finalized. The patient accepts the aesthetic aspects of the restoration. This visit usually has a duration of between two and four hours but could be longer depending on technical aspects and patient co-operation.
9. The restoration is ready for temporary cementation for a period of one or two weeks to verify function, soft tissue response, comfort and aesthetic acceptability. Final cementation follows if no further adjustments are required.		

* See chapter 5

Table 1 A typical arrangement for a patient requiring an aesthetic restoration.

2.3 Protocol for the Technician

Technicians who are committed to the highest aesthetic standards must be prepared to view each case as an individual and not as a number of work units. The role of the technician should be to provide the optimal restoration and with this responsibility should be prepared, where necessary, to implement additional procedures such as trial wax crowns or alternative laboratory techniques to achieve the desired result.

Traditional practice usually means that patients do not see the technician responsible for the aesthetic result expected. Even when a meeting is arranged, it is usually of .such short duration that the technician is expected to make the colour selection in one visit of perhaps 10 minutes.

Technicians are often requested to attend the dental surgery and make colour selections or alter a restoration. It is in these circumstances that technicians are severely handicapped. Ideally the technician should have unrestricted access to the patient within the laboratory environment, as it is in this way that artistic creativity is fulfilled without constraints such as unfamiliar surroundings, lighting and equipment.

Alterations and colour adjustments can be carried out with the benefit of direct access to the patient, providing an opportunity to create the ideal technical and aesthetic restoration.

For this to happen dentists must have complete confidence in their technician's ability and accept a degree of delegation over the aesthetic control.

Laboratory procedures

Patients need to be received in the most professional environment possible. A separate room with lighting designed for shade selection and equipped to make alterations to ceramic work is desirable, especially for the comfort and privacy of the patient. Surgical gloves should be worn and an air of professionalism must prevail. Every effort should be made to make the visit as relaxed and pleasant for the patient as possible.

Provided the patient has been informed of the necessary procedures, no inconvenience will be too much, as all effort is directed towards benefiting the patient. Therefore, if preparatory ground work has been laid, a more successful outcome is likely to result.

Figs 57 and 58 General views of the Korson laboratory illustrate the professional environment necessary for patient and dentist to feel confident.

Fig 57

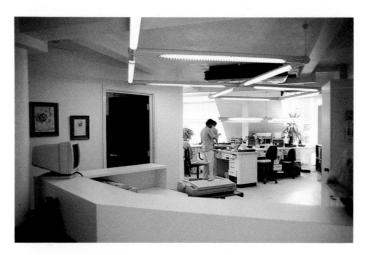

Fig 58

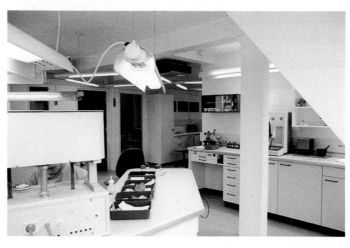

Figs 59 and 60 Reception/ office area.

Fig 59

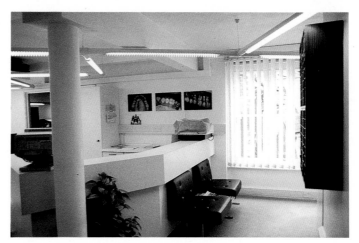

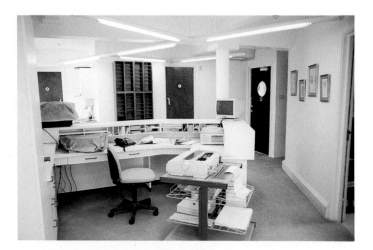

Fig 60

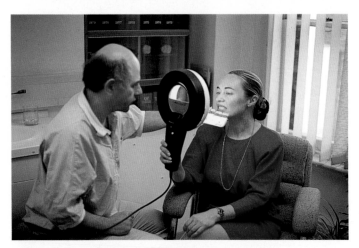

Fig 61 Shade selection takes place in a specially prepared room affording the patient a degree of privacy.

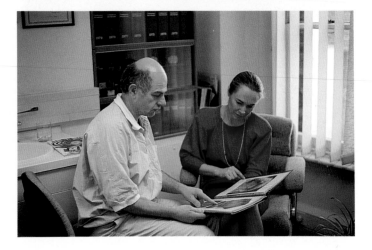

Fig 62 The patient and the author in discussion during the initial visit.

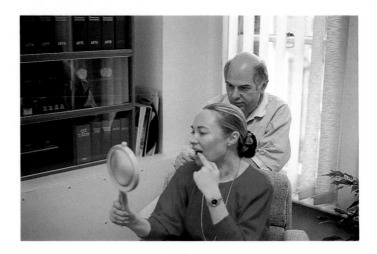

Fig 63 Taking a position behind the patient will provide the same view as the patient's own. This can be a valuable aid when observation of subtle nuances in shape and position are required.

2.4 Involvement of the Patient

For such a relationship to exist between the patient and dentist/technician team a high degree of commitment is required. Not every person attending the dental surgery for treatment will be receptive to this, therefore, an assessment should take place by the dental surgeon to ascertain the likely response to this special relationship. Acceptability by the patient may be influenced by:

a) Ability to pay
b) Available time
c) Patient perception of their appearance
d) Travel distance

Once the patient has been educated to appreciate the clinical and technical expertise and effort required and has accepted the necessary involvement, they will willingly become part of 'the team'.

Working in this way an understanding of the artistry and associated technical problems experienced by the dental technician will prevail, allowing the technician complete freedom to take photographs, fabricate sample tabs, aesthetic wax trials, bisque trials and if necessary, start again.

2.5 Technical Procedures with Patient Involvement at the Laboratory

For optimal results the following laboratory visits have been recommended and are summarized as:

First visit   Initial shade selection

Second visit   Aesthetic wax trial

Third visit   Ceramic bisque trial and completion of restoration

First visit

Initial shade selection

During this visit the initial shade selection is made. Photographs are taken and if necessary custom tabs are fabricated. The patient's expectations are discussed.

Many people are unused to this form of treatment, therefore, the reason for further visits and the expected time that these will take is explained.

Second visit

Aesthetic wax trial

The aesthetic wax trial is tried in and form and position are checked for aesthetic acceptability. Harmony with tissue contour is verified and if necessary adjustments to the wax are easily carried out to achieve the desired result.

Contra Indications

Anterior guidance cannot be checked at this stage as the wax is too fragile to withstand heavy occlusal function. Aesthetic waxes are not suitable for shade analysis.

Third visit

Ceramic bisque trial and completion of restoration

Even though the aesthetic wax diagnostic stage has been simulated in the ceramic, a bisque trial is essential as final adjustments to contour and position may still be necessary and final colour adjustments will also be required.

The restoration is viewed under magnification, as it is only in this way that the refining of delicate anatomy is achieved. Incisal edge shape should be in harmony with neighbouring dentition, including such characteristics as developmental lobes and associated lamellae, wear facets and chipped enamel. Surface detail such as ridge and groove patterns as well as surface perikymata must all be observed and simulated on the restoration.

Staining procedures

The restoration is placed on the preparation and lip retractors are used to provide easy access. It is dried and surface staining procedures are employed. However, staining is limited to minor characterisation rather than major alterations in shade, generally such alterations require the further addition of porcelain or a complete remake. The patient may view the restoration in the Waldmann Colorident lamp.*

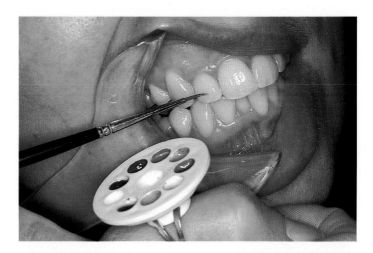

Fig 64 Intraoral staining. Note lip retractors are used to provide easy access to the restoration.

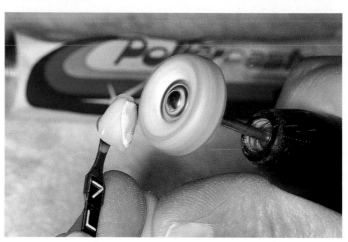

Fig 65 If required, diamond or Universal polishing paste is used to achieve a high lustre.

Following glaze cycle, the restoration is checked to ensure surface texture is in harmony with the remaining dentition. Surface polishing of the porcelain to achieve the correct degree of lustre is carried out with pumice and a felt wheel and where a high lustre is required further polishing with Universal polishing paste is undertaken.** (fig 65)

One week post cementation

A photograph session is planned for one week after cementation, following tissue recovery.

* Waldmann, D-7730 Villingen-Schwenningen, Germany.

**Ivoclar, Schaan, Leichtenstein.

2.6 Dentist — Technician Communication when the Patient is Unable to Visit the Technician

Occasions arise when patients are unable to make visits to the technician. Even in these circumstances many of the techniques advocated are still relevant.

Procedures the technician would normally carry out can, with suitable liaison between dentist and technician, be successfully executed by the dental surgeon.

Techniques to relay information for aesthetic requirements to the technician should include:*

At impression stage

1. Intraoral photographs of:**
a) Oral situation prior to treatment
b) Shade tabs adjacent to teeth
   Intraoral photographs of shade tabs should include:
   General colour with 'custom guide'
   High chroma areas such as root, neck, and occlusal fossa shown with the 'custom guide' or the relative commercial shade guide
   Enamel colour with enamel guide
   Texture and lustre guides

c) Temporary restoration.
2. Study cast of dentition prior to treatment
3. Cast of temporary restoration.
4. An indication of desired characterization, for middle-aged and aged dentition.
5. Patient's expectation in relation to aesthetic requirements.

Ceramic bisque trial stage

The bisque trial is tried in and checked for the following:

1. Accuracy in centric occlusion
2. Posterior disclusion/group function
3. Anterior guidance
4. Speech function
5. Marginal accuracy
6. Compatibility with soft tissues
7. Contact areas between teeth
8. Emergence profile
9. Aesthetic acceptability

It is important that where discrepancies are found in either occlusion or marginal accuracy that the restoration is checked on the working casts and dies to try and establish the cause for future reference.

After all checks are finalized and the restoration is satisfactory, any aesthetic adjustments need to be conveyed to the technician. Various methods are available to achieve this.

---

* It is beyond the scope of this book to describe techniques other than those required to achieve aesthetic harmony.

** See Section 6.4 Communication Through Photography.

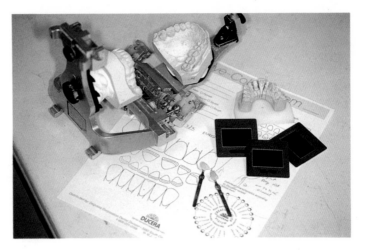

Fig 66 Records to convey aesthetic information to the technician should include shade prescription, photographs, study casts and various shade guides.

Alteration to contour or position

The dental surgeon may adjust the porcelain by grinding and where additions are required tooth coloured waxes are used to indicate the appearance. Should the axis of the teeth be incorrect, pencil lines indicating the correct axis are marked upon the ceramic. Photographs should be taken both before adjustment and after. Colour of the bisque ceramic may be improved in the photograph by the application of ceramic stain fluid or glycerine upon the surface. If extensive alterations are necessary, a retry should be arranged.

Cementation

Many surgeons fit the restoration with temporary cement to allow the patient time to accept the restoration and to be sure that it functions correctly. Following a suitable waiting period the restoration is cemented permanently. Photographs of the restoration and of tissue response may be taken at the visit, prior to removal of the temporary cemented restoration.

Photographs of the final result are invaluable as a learning experience. Slide transparencies projected upon a large screen provide valuable information. Joint discussion will help with better assessments for the future. Photographs should include those advocated under wax and bisque trials.

3 Tissue Management for Aesthetic and Biological Harmony

A. C. S. Druttman M.Sc. B.Ch.D.

The use of ceramic materials in the replacement of tooth structure should not only emulate the natural tooth, but should also be placed in an environment of biological harmony. This means that the natural contour of the tooth, and its relationship to the surrounding soft tissue have to be understood and respected.

Success of the final result can only be achieved when there is an understanding between the dentist and the technician of each others' roles in the execution of their work. All too often, when clinical or laboratory procedures are carried out inadequately, each blames the other for the failure.

The purpose of this chapter is to describe to technicians and dentists alike, clinical procedures which are used successfully to obtain aesthetic results in a healthy soft tissue environment. It is by definition subjective, but has been based on sound principles established in the literature.

Careful treatment planning, precise clinical and laboratory techniques and close co-operation between all those involved will give the best opportunity to achieve a pleasing result.

3.1 Preparation Design

Placement of margins

Margin placement has to be considered carefully in the preparation design, as it may well influence the health of the adjacent periodontal tissues. Even well fitting restorations with subgingival margins are more likely to produce gingivitis than those with supragingival margins. (Renggli and Regolati, 1972) Positioning of the preparation margin will depend on such factors as the patient's smile line, caries, resorption, fractures, crown length and abrasion cavities.

Supragingival margins may be acceptable in the anterior region of the mouth, depending on such factors as smile line (fig 67) and susceptibility to periodontal disease. It should, however, be planned and discussed with the patient, rather than inflicted as a *fait accompli.* Where supragingival margins are contraindicated, they can be located at the free gingival margin (fig 68) without significant increase in gingivitis. (Valderhaug, 1980, Muller, 1986) The placement of margins subgingivally requires very careful consideration. Not only is assessment of fit more difficult (Zander, 1957), but maintenance of healthy tissues around subgingival margins is considerably more difficult than supragingival margins (Silness, 1970) and there can be no guarantee that the relationship of the gingiva to the margin will maintain itself. (Kennedy, 1990)

Tooth reduction

The ability of the technician to achieve an optimal aesthetic result depends on the adequate removal of tooth substance. The dentist is often faced with a dilemma. Inadequate removal may lead to an overcontoured crown or insufficient space to mask the opaque layer of porcelain. In either case this may lead to poor aesthetics. Yet excess removal may compromise retention, the strength of the underlying core and the vitality or viability of the pulp.

The recommended reduction of labial tooth substance for a bonded porcelain crown is 1.5mm. This can be facilitated by cutting depth grooves in the enamel at the start of preparation. It can be further verified by measuring the thickness of the labial aspect of the provisional restoration.

Fit and marginal finish

The quality of the marginal finish of the preparation can affect not only the fit of the restoration, but also the soft tissue response, especially in the case of subgingival restorations. Indeed Richter and Ueno (1973) suggested that fit was more important than the position of the margin when considering the soft tissue response. Regardless of the type of marginal finish, the purpose should be to produce a smooth margin (fig 69) which the technician is able to identify clearly and finish to without difficulty. If the margin is rough or indistinct, it will be more difficult for the technician to determine the finish line and, therefore, to produce a restoration that fits accurately. This may cause an increase in plaque accumulation and consequently cause microleakage of bacteria and the ultimate failure of the restoration.

Smooth margins can be achieved in a number of different ways. After preparation with diamond burs, the procedure may be finished with matching smooth grit diamonds, tungsten carbide or stone finishing burs. The author's preference is to use coarse grit diamond burs for the initial

48

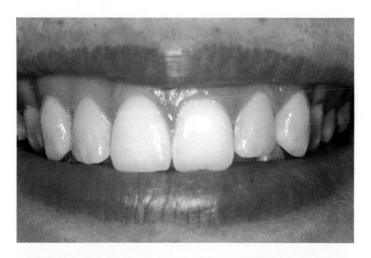

Fig 67 A natural smile showing the gingival margin.

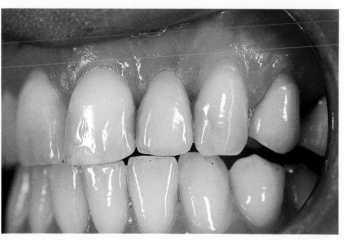

Fig 68 Metal-ceramic crown on the left lateral incisor, preparation margin at the free gingival margin.

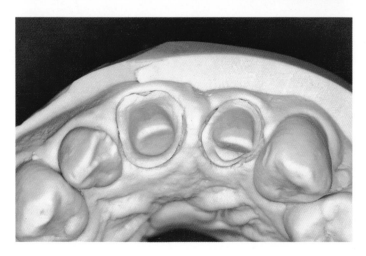

Fig 69 A smooth finish is particularly important when preparing for a porcelain butt fit on the labial shoulder.

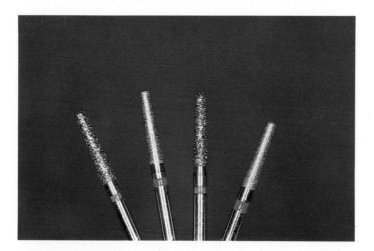

Fig 70 Course grit burs (125μm) and equivalent fine grit burs (30μm) for crown preparation.

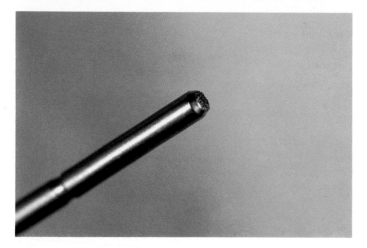

Fig 71 End cutting bur with a rounded edge for finishing shoulder preparations.

preparation, followed by the equivalent fine grit burs* to complete the preparation (fig 70). Shoulders for porcelain butt fits are finished with a diamond end cutting bur,** which have a rounded edge so as not to create steps in the preparation (fig 71).

* GERB. Brasseler GmbH & Co, KG, D-4920 Lemgo, Germany.

** Premier Dental Products Co., Norristown PA 19401, USA.

3.2 Care of the soft tissues

Management of the gingival tissues is no less important than the careful preparation of the tooth. Aesthetic porcelain work can easily be spoilt by an adverse soft tissue response.

Careful management of the soft tissues is important for the following reasons:

1. Predictable position of the gingival margin post operatively.
2. Greater ease in achieving an accurate impression because of reduced crevicular exudate. This leads to improved fit of final restorations and hence, long-term periodontal health.
3. Greater ease in achieving accurate provisional restorations.

The gingivae can be damaged by plaque accumulation through poor oral hygiene measures, badly fitting restorations or a combination of both. They can be further traumatized during preparation, impression procedures and temporization.

Care of the tissues before preparation

Prior to any definitive operative procedures, the soft tissues should be rendered healthy. Any pre-existing restorations which may prejudice the health of the adjacent soft tissues should be re-shaped or replaced to facilitate home-care procedures. Ill fitting crowns and bridges (figs 72 and 73) should be replaced with provisional units which would facilitate tissue healing (fig 74). If the margins of these restorations violate the attachment apparatus, it may be advisable to consider periodontal surgical procedures to produce a more favourable relationship with the gingivae. However, this may destroy the interdental papillae and have a deleterious effect on the final aesthetic result. This has to be considered at the planning stage. Provided that the attachment apparatus has not been violated, careful subgingival preparation may produce a more aesthetically pleasing result (fig 75) although this is likely to put greater demands on the dentist's skills and the patient's plaque control.

Care of the tissues during preparation

A careful preparation technique adjacent to healthy gingivae should produce minimal damage to the soft tissues (fig 76). This requires the use of the appropriately shaped bur for each situation. Wherever possible margins should be left supragingival, as this will reduce the potential for soft tissue laceration and facilitate impression procedures. If the gingival margin is damaged or inflamed it may be prudent to delay the impression until healing has occurred. (Aneroth and Goransson 1965)

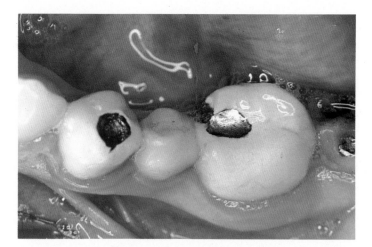

Fig 72 Ill fitting three unit bridge, note the darker colour of the inflamed gingivae and the rolled margin.

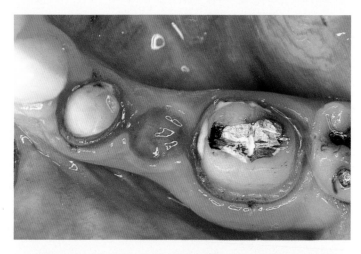

Fig 73 The gingival condition is seen more clearly after removal of the bridge.

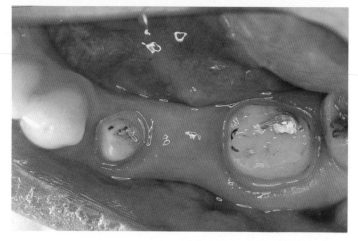

Fig 74 The gingivae have improved considerably after electrosurgical removal of soft tissue, repreparation and temporisation.

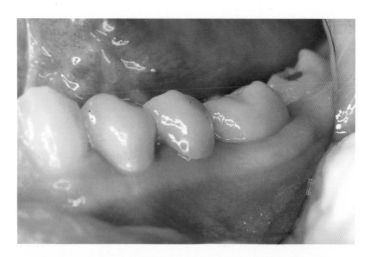

Fig 75 The final restoration, note the improved appearance of the gingivae.

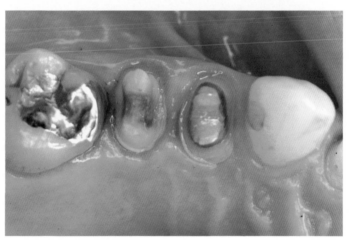

Fig 76 A careful preparation technique should produce minimal trauma to the gingival tissues.

3.3 Preparing for the Impression

Retraction cord

To ensure the production of an accurate impression, the finishing line must be adequately exposed. Where the preparation is finished at or below the free gingival margin, it is advisable to use retraction cord (fig 77). The purpose of this measure is to temporarily displace the gingiva from the tooth. The impression material can then be flowed beyond the margin of the preparation to enable the finishing line and the root shape beyond to be recorded. The haemostatic chemicals in the cord help to control any seepage of blood or exudate from the gingival crevice.

The size of cord chosen should be related to the dimensions of the gingival crevice. If the cord is too large it is likely to spring out from the crevice, if it is too small or is placed too deeply into the crevice, the gingiva may collapse over the cord and inadequate retraction will be achieved. Where there is a deep gingival sulcus, a double cord technique can be used. Cord of a narrow diameter is first placed into the sulcus and followed by the insertion of a thicker cord. The second cord is then removed while the first is left in place for the impression.

Great care must be used to place the cord. Only sufficient pressure to hold it in place should be used. Greater force may strip the attached gingiva from the cementum and cause gingival recession.

Electrosurgery

There are situations where the gingival tissues cannot be managed with cord alone. Badly fitting restorations or caries may cause tissue to become inflamed or hyperplastic and in these situations hemorrhage from the marginal gingivae can easily distort the impression. Electrosurgery may be used to remove any excess soft tissue. Different sizes and shapes of tips* (fig 78) allow for very accurate control of soft tissue removal (fig 79). The margins of the preparation can be

*Ellman International Manufacturing Inc. Hewlett NY 11557 USA

readily exposed to enable a well fitting provisional restoration to be made. When the position of the gingival margin is critical, final impressions can be postponed until the tissues have healed.

Electrosurgery may be helpful, even with healthy tissues where there is little gingival crevice. Minimal tissue removal, (fig 80) followed by the use of retraction cord enables the dentist to produce clear impressions. From these the technician can produce models where the margins are clearly visible and the possibility of errors in trimming the dies is minimized.

Careful use of electrosurgery in the superficial part of the gingival crevice results in little, if any, residual damage to the gingivae. (Coelho, Cavallaro and Rothschild 1975) However, abuse can cause severe periodontal destruction. (O'Leary, Standish and Bloomer, 1973) Pameijer (1985) suggested that only fully filtered and rectified current should be used from a unit that has a high frequency output (4MHz). This would certainly be the case around teeth where the soft tissues may be thin and fragile and tissue shrinkage should be minimized. A fully rectified current can be used where cutting with haemostasis is required and where tissue shrinkage is less critical (Sherman 1992) the tip should enter the soft tissues to a depth of no more than one millimetre, as regeneration of the soft tissues is adversely affected by the amount of tissue removed. (Coelho, Cavallaro and

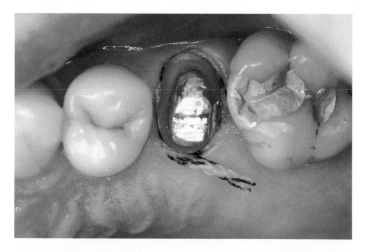

Fig 77 Retraction cord in place, note the condition of the gingival tissues.

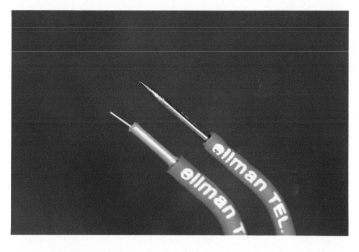

Fig 78 Electrosurgery tips, No 118 for anterior teeth where tissue shrinkage should be minimized (left) No 113F where tissue shrinkage is less critical (right).

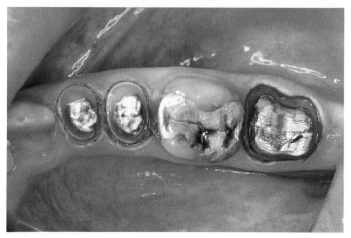

Fig 79 Exposure of the gingival margin using electrosurgery.

55

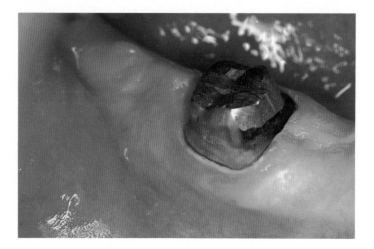

Fig 80 Minimal soft tissue removal to facilitate identification of the preparation margin.

Rothschild, 1975). Where the aesthetics are of prime importance, as on the labial aspect of anterior teeth, it may be advisable to avoid electrosurgery.

3.4 Impression Procedures

Many modern impression materials are highly accurate if used correctly. Inaccuracies that occur in the clinical situation are usually due to inadequacies of technique. Choice will depend on personal preference.

The author's preference is for reversible hydrocolloid for the following reasons:

1. The material is hydrophyllic (made up of 80% water). It, there-fore, will give an accurate impression, not only of the preparation itself (fig 81), but of the whole arch without the need to maintain a dry field.

2. Special trays are not required and the stock metal trays provided have excellent rigidity.

3. The impression material conditions the gingival tissues so that improved results can be obtained with repeated impressions.

4. The system is clean and the impressions are very easy to pour. Casts are easy to remove after the stone has set because of the low rigidity of the gelled hydrocolloid.

5. The cost of the hydrocolloid impression material is lower than other materials.

There are, however, certain disadvantages which the dentist has to be aware of.

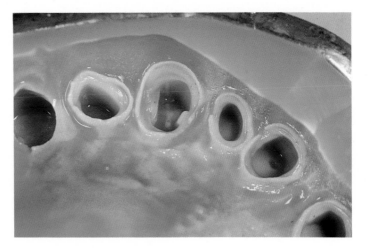

Fig 81 Hydrocolloid impression after electrosurgery and retraction cord have been used.

1. Impressions have to be poured up within a short time, so either the laboratory has to be close by or the impressions must be poured up at the surgery. This will require access to a vacuum mixer and a vibrator. A small vacuum pump and a Bego** hand mixing bowl are economical alternatives to laboratory vacuum mixers.
2. The capital costs of the hydrocolloid conditioning unit, trays and accessories are high.
3. The shear strength is lower than rubber base materials and in thin sections, that is, in the gingival sulcus, the material may tear and cause difficulty in reading the margin.
4. Impressions cannot be electroplated.

** Bremer Goldschlagerei Wilh Herbst, Emil Sommer Str.7, Postfach 410162, D-2800 Bremen 41, Germany.

Accurate impressions can also be made using rubber based materials, but it is imperative to keep the preparations and soft tissues dry (fig 82).

3.5 Fabrication of Provisional Restorations

The provisional restoration plays an important role in restorative procedures. Certain requirements should be fulfilled by the provisional restorations. These include protection of the pulp, maintenance of periodontal health, maintenance of occlusal stability and adequate durability. They can also be invaluable in giving diagnostic information which can be used in the manufacture of the definitive restorations.

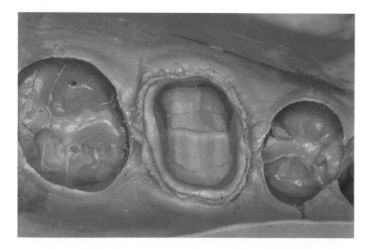

Fig 82 Rubber based materials have many advantages and are highly accurate when used correctly.

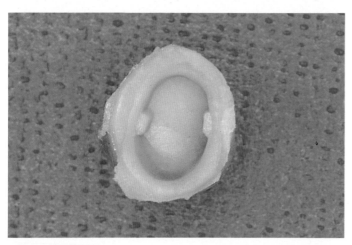

Fig 83 Provisional acrylic restoration, note the clearly identifiable margin.

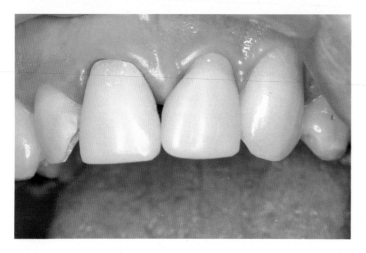

Fig 84 Provisional restorations on the upper left central and right lateral incisors.

Lack of care at this stage can cause periodontal inflammation and gingival recession. (Donaldson, 1973) Achieving an accurate fit and correct contours in the provisional restorations is an exacting and time-consuming procedure and sadly, is often neglected. It will, however, allow gingival tissues to recover rapidly from the effects of operative procedures and inadequacies of previous restorations.

A clearly identifiable preparation margin will facilitate the manufacture of an accurate provisional crown or bridge (fig 83) and it may be advisable to use retraction cord or electrosurgery to expose the margins of the preparation, even if impression procedures are delayed.

An accurate fit can be obtained with any of the accepted methods of making provisional restorations. Use of the currently available materials permits reline and addition to ensure correct fit and contour. Provisional units should be carefully finished and polished. If they will be in place for more than a few days, the contour fit and finish should resemble that of the final restoration. (Kennedy, 1990)

The gingival response to the contour of the provisional restorations can also be used as a guide for the shape of the final restorations (fig 84). They may also be used during periodontal therapy to improve the gingival condition, prior to taking impressions for the final restorations.

3.6 Crown Contour at the Margin

Inadequate reduction in the preparation for full crowns often leads to overcontouring of restorations. A study by Parkinson (1976) showed that 80% of full gold crowns of those sampled were wider than the original tooth and of the porcelain fused to metal crowns, all were too wide buccolingually. Whenever possible the cervical contours of the crown should be flat or even slightly concave. (Jameson & Malone 1982)

The term emergence profile has been used and is defined as the contour of the restoration at the point of emergence from the gingival sulcus. (Stein & Kuwata, 1977) The benefit of a flat emergence profile (fig 85) is easier cleaning of the cervical area and consequently, a better gingival response. This particularly applies to proximal as well as buccal and lingual contours. Overcontouring is a significant factor in gingival inflammation. (Perel 1971) Crown shape should facilitate normal home-care procedures for the removal of plaque. Interproximal spaces should, if at all possible, be large enough to allow the use of either floss or interspace brushes.

Adequate tooth reduction at the margin will allow the technician to produce an aesthetic crown without overcontouring. The provisional restoration can give a very good indica-

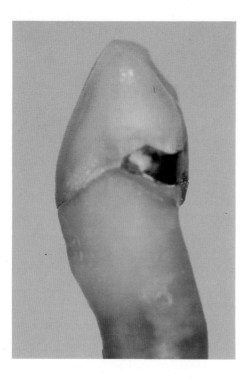

tion of the gingival response to the shape of the final restoration. Any blanching of the gingival tissues when the provisional crown is inserted will indicate where it is overcontoured. The emergence profile can be easily altered and a biologically harmonious contour can be established. A bisque stage try-in of the final restoration will allow the gingival tissue response to be assessed after the gingivae have recovered from the impression procedure and the emergence profile altered if necessary.

Fig 85 Flat emergence profile on the labial aspect of the crown.

References

1. *Aneroth G. & Goransson P:* Exposing the gingival margin by taking impressions with elastic materials — some clinical and histopathological aspects. Odont Revy 73: 394, 1965.
2. *Coelho D. H., Cavallaro J. & Rothschild E. A:* Gingival recession with electrosurgery for impression making. J Prosth Dent 33: 422, 1975.
3. *Donaldson D:* The aetiology of gingival recession associated with temporary crowns. J Periodontol 44: 691, 1973.
4. *Kennedy E. B:* In Glickman's Clinical Periodontol: 924 7th ed. 1990 W. B. Saunders & Co. Philadelphia, USA.
5. *Muller H. P:* The effect of artificial crown margins at the gingival margin on the periodontal conditions in a group of periodontally supervised patients treated with fixed bridges. J Clinical Periodontol 13: 97-102, 1986.
6. *O'Leary T. J., Standish S. M. & Bloomer R. S:* Severe periodontal destruction following impression procedures. J Periodontol 44: 43-48, 1973.
7. *Pameijer J. H:* Periodontal and occlusal factors in crown and bridge procedures. Dental Centre for Postgraduate Courses, Amsterdam, 1985.
8. *Parkinson C. F:* Excessive crown contours facilitate endemic plaque niches. J Prosth Dent 35: 424, 1976.
9. *Perel M:* Axial crown contours. J Prosth Dent 25: 642, 1971.
10. *Renggli H. H. & Regolati B:* Gingival inflammation and plaque accumulation by well adapted supragingival and subgingival provisional restorations. Helv Odonto Acta 16: 1972.
11. *Richter W. A. & Ueno H:* Relationship of crown margin placement to gingival inflammation. J Prosthet Dent 30: 156, 1973.
12. *Sherman J. A:* Oral electrosurgery an illustrated clinical guide, Martin Dunitz, London, 1992.
13. *Silness J:* Periodontal conditions in patients treated with dental bridges. III The relationship between the location of the crown margins and the periodontal condition. J Periodont Res 5: 225, 1974.
14. *Stein R. S. & Kuwata M:* A dentist and a dental technologist analyse current ceramo-metal procedures. Dent Clin Am 21: 729, 1977.
15. *Valderhaug J:* Periodontal conditions and carious lesions following the insertion of fixed prostheses: a 10 year follow-up study. Internat Dent J 30: 296, 1980.
16. *Zander H. A:* Effect of silicate and amalgam on gingiva. J Am Dent Assoc 55: 11, 1957.

4 Impressions and Occlusal Records

The accuracy of impressions and occlusal records and the way in which these are handled has a direct bearing upon the transfer of information from the oral situation to the working casts and their articulation. This chapter suggests a working practise to maintain optimal accuracy and replication of the oral situation.

4.1 Impressions and Die Trimming

Impressions should be inspected under magnification by the dentist and again upon receipt by the laboratory.

It is assumed that a minimum standard is one in which the preparation margin is clearly visible in all areas and there are no obvious defects. Impressions of full coverage crown preparations need to extend beyond the prepared margin by 1-2mm, this will enable the crown contour to be contiguous with emergence profile. Failure to do this will cause crowns to be either under or more often, over-contoured. (Martignini and Schoenenburg, 1990)

Regions of the mouth where aesthetics are a factor require specific shoulder margin design. When aesthetics are not of prime concern bevelled shoulders or chamfer margins are advocated, mainly due to the geometry of these designs which minimise errors upon cementation. (Shillingburg, Hobbs, Fisher, 1973. Rosner, 1963. Kuwata, 1986.)

To achieve an optimal fit margins should be clearly defined, any small steps or other surface irregularities such as fine chipping of the enamel rods at the preparation edge must be avoided. This will create problems for the ceramic margin to adapt with complete integrity.

Adequate shoulder width is important to prevent reflective opaque layers showing through the overlying dentine and enamel porcelain, with 90° shoulders prepared to maximize strength of edge porcelain.

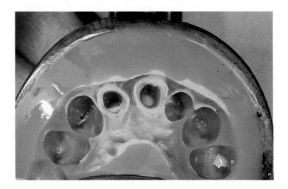

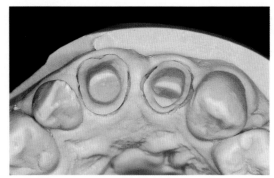

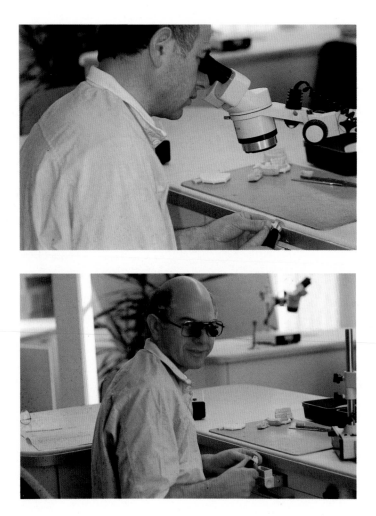

Fig 86 The impression should be as near perfect an imprint of the tooth preparation as possible. Hydrocolloid impression fulfills all the necessary criteria (dentist, A. Druttman).

Fig 87 Cast demonstrates an extension beyond the tooth preparation. This will aid in establishing a correct physiologic contour from tooth structures to the restoration.

Fig 88 The stereo microscope* provides a clear image. However, it has limited mobility and requires working under a fixed position. In addition, depth of field is limited.

Fig 89 Keeler Loupes** are more convenient, although of small magnification (between x two - x four) they have a high resolution.

* Prior S2000. Prior James Swift, Fulbourn, Cambridge.

** Keeler Ltd. Clewer Hill Road, Windsor, Berks S44 4AA.

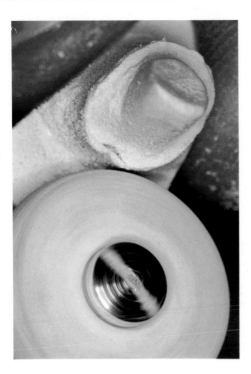

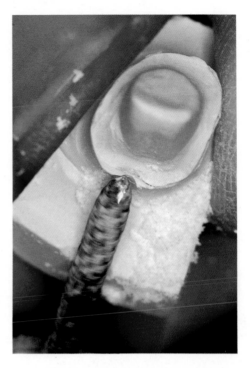

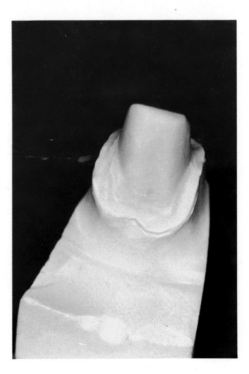

Fig 90 Grey silicone rubber wheels are used to fine trim excess plaster. This stage is executed under stereo microscopy.

Fig 91 Multifluted carbide bur is employed to trim into the furcation.

Fig 92 The completed trimmed die. Note that irrespective of where the finish margin of the preparation is, the die is only trimmed as far as the impression of tooth structure. The shoulder preparation must be smooth and without irregularities which can cause problems for porcelain adaptation.

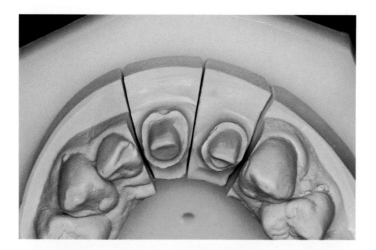

Figs 93 and 94 Assembled dies on the working cast.

Fig 93

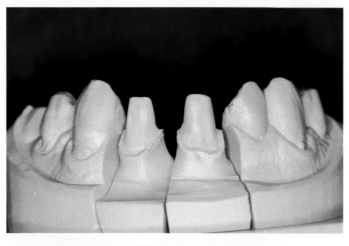

Fig 94

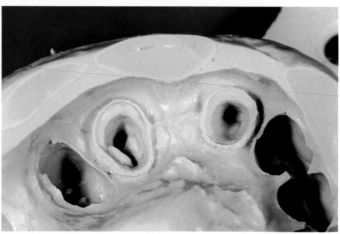

Fig 95 Excellent results are possible with Addition Cured Silicone (dentist, S. Selwyn).

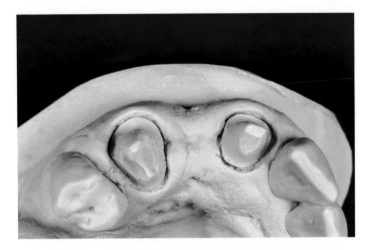

Fig 96 Stone cast resulting from silicone impression.

Figs 97 and 98 It is important that the shoulder preparation extends into the interproximal area at least half way between labial and palatal, if aesthetic margins are required.

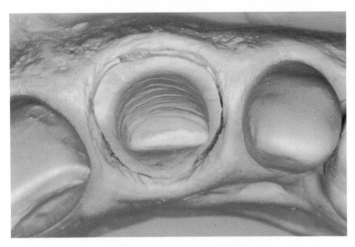

Fig 97

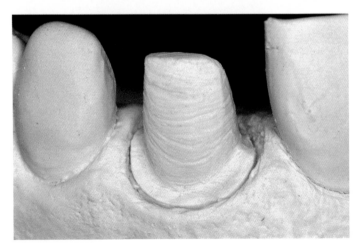

Fig 98

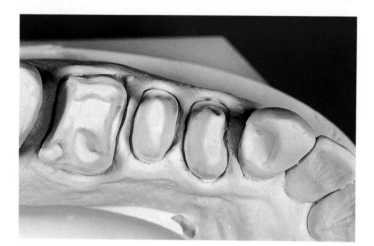

Fig 99 Preparations for metal ceramic crowns on maxillary bi-cuspids. It is not necessary to extend the shoulder into the interproximal at the distal aspect as this will be hidden from view. However, if aesthetics are a factor the shoulder width should be extended into the mesial interproximal region.

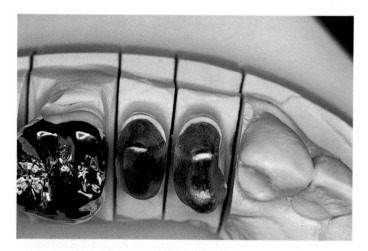

Fig 100 Metal substrate design.

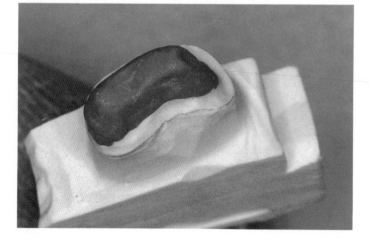

Fig 101 Close detail of first bi-cuspid mesial shoulder is not well defined and appears as a shallow chamfer preparation in this area.

Fig 102 Close detail of the metal substrate illustrates the problem, there is insufficient width to create depth of porcelain in this region. The result will seem to be adequate when viewed on the cast, but will appear bright in the mouth. This is a common mistake and most frequently occurs in canine teeth, as they are the first to start the rotation in the dental arch it is critical that the shoulder width is continued into the interproximal area, ensuring any metal is completely hidden from view.

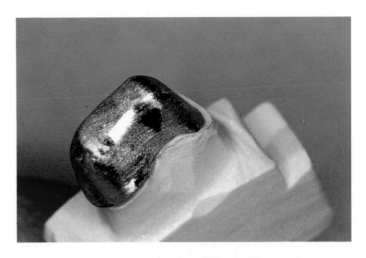

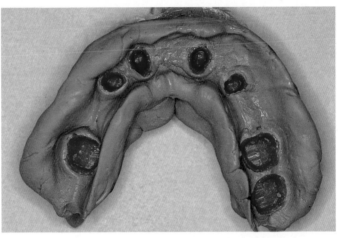

Fig 103 DuraLay impression copings in the pick-up impression.

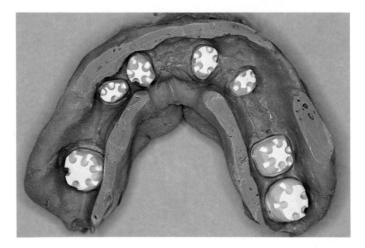

Fig 104 Stone dies are waxed into position prior to pouring the working cast.

Multiple Abutment Impression Techniques

In multiple abutment situations difficulties may arise in capturing the complete detail of every abutment. If this is a problem several impressions are taken, concentrating on achieving a good impression of each abutment. Dies are poured and trimmed, Dura-Lay* copings are fabricated and returned to the operator for seating upon the abutments prior to a pick-up impression. The accuracy of the individual dies can also be checked using this technique (Figs 103 and 104).

Faults in impression technique can generate complications in occlusion. Many of these appear to emanate from two stage techniques, incomplete impressions or quadrant impressions. Impressions which have lifted

* Reliance Dental Manufacturing Co, Worth, Illinois 60482.

away from the impression tray create an exaggerated curve of Von Spey with consequential occlusal distortion. Opposing arch alginate impressions are often considered less important and, therefore, the possibility of inaccuracy increases.

Optimal intercuspation of the articulated casts

Minor occlusal inaccuracies in the cast can often be rectified by marking the high spots with double sided articulating foil, premature contacts due to false or indistinct fossae detail will show quite clearly, adjustment of these areas by trimming allows closer intercuspation. Contact of wear facets are verified with Shimstock.

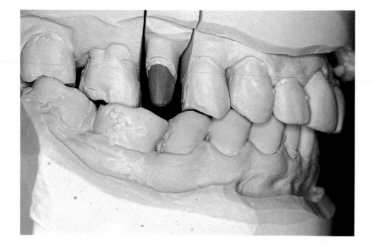

Fig 105 Casts show premature contact in the molar region and an opening between the second bi-cuspids due to lifting of the opposing arch alginate impression from the impression tray.

Figs 106 and 107 Occlusal markings disclose premature contacts due to distortion.

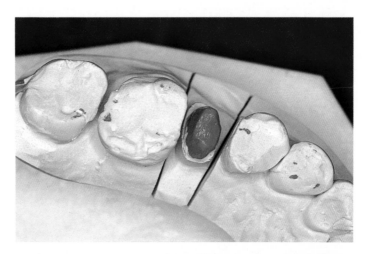

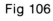
Fig 106

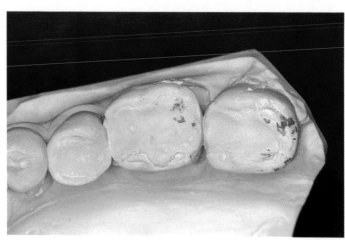

Fig 107

Fig 108 After adjustments by spot grinding the teeth occlude.

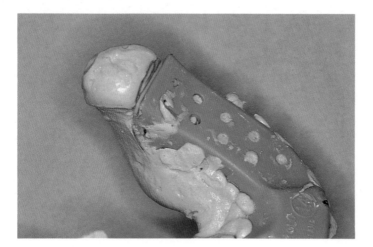

Fig 109 Alginate impression has lifted away from the impression tray, causing inaccuracy in occlusion.

Impressions

Impressions must be completely supported by the impression tray, often the last molar is beyond the distal extension of the tray, the possible distortion in this region will cause discrepancies in occlusion. Technicians should be aware that casts with open contacts between wear facets indicate the likely distortion caused from unsupported impressions.

4.2 Occlusal Records

This is an area which in the laboratory presents the highest percentage of discrepancy and liaison is important if occlusal schemes are to be realised. Records taken in centric occlusion should be marked accordingly, as should those taken in centric relation. If the technician does not realise a record in centric relation has been recorded, he is likely to assume it is an incorrect record of centric occlusion.

Occlusal records taken over terminal abutments, or where there is a lack of opposing posterior contacts to use as a reference must encompass the preparations, so that location onto the master cast is accurate. Occlusal records taken before preparation of the teeth or over temporary crowns can cause problems in locating the record accurately on the cast.

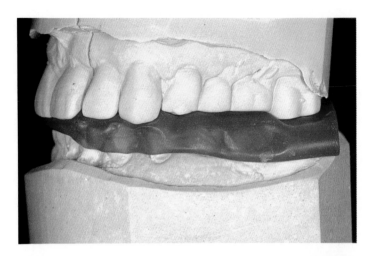

Fig 110 Intraoral wax registration of centric occlusion. Full intercuspation of the dentition and accurate seating of casts into the registration are hidden from view, causing possible inaccuracies.

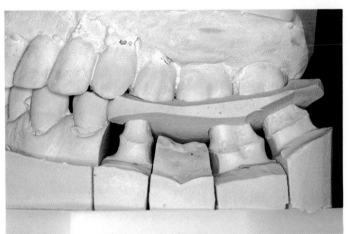

Fig 111 Occlusãl record is sectioned to observe that the cast is completely seated.*

* Verone Putty. Davis Schottlander & Davis Ltd, Letchworth, Herts, England.

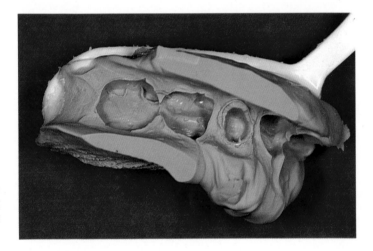

Fig 112 Sectional impression provides little information about cross arch occlusion or tooth contour.

The registration should be sectioned to ensure complete intercuspation and to facilitate removal of all soft tissue contacts. This technique could be usefully employed in the surgery during registration, in those cases where the existing occlusal relationship is to be maintained and where there are sufficient occlusal contacts in the remaining dentition to verify full intercuspation.

Records confined to the prepared teeth are acceptable, however, care must be taken to ensure that complete intercuspation has been achieved in the remaining dentition, as any opening of contacts will cause a discrepancy between those areas and that of the record.

Casts are adjusted until complete intercuspation has occured and wear facets correspond with centric occlusion and excursive movements.

Liaison with the dentist should indicate where Shimstock contacts occur and movements on the articulator correspond to those in the mouth. After mounting, the articulation should be returned to the clinician for verification of centric occlusion/relation and excursive movements.

Incomplete impressions of the dental arch cause various difficulties:

1. Inaccurate mounting of casts as tilting occurs.
2. Non-working side disclusion cannot be verified.
3. Opposing side anatomy is lost. (Full arch pre-operative alginate impressions would remedy this factor.)

It is recommended that sectional impressions are only used as part of an overall technique, which will ultimately result in a full arch cast, for example, transfer copings or the transference of the restoration to a full arch cast for final occlusal adjustments.

References

1. *Kuwata M:* Colour Atlas of Ceramo-Metal Technology. Ishiyaku Euro America, Inc. pp34-38 1986.
2. *Martignini & Sheonenburg:* Precision Fixed Prosthodontics: Clinical and Laboratory Aspects. Quintessence Pub. Co. Inc. Chicago. Illinois. pp53-56 1990.
3. *Rosner D:* Function, placement and reproduction at bevels for gold castings. J. Pros. Dent 13 1160-1166 Nov. 1963.
4. *Shillingburg H. Hobo S. & Fisher D. W:* Preparation design and margin distortion in porcelain-fused-to-metal restorations. J. Pros. Dent. 29, 276-284 1973.

5   Aesthetic Wax Diagnostic Control

This chapter provides information on waxing techniques which will impart a high degree of visual conception prior to the definitive technical construction, thereby allowing the dentist, dental technician and patient a better control of aesthetics.

5.1 Reasons for Aesthetic Wax Studies

Many times the question is asked 'What shape are my new teeth going to be?' or 'How do you know what shape to make my teeth?'

Often patients requiring extensive anterior restorations wish to have the opportunity to envisage the anticipated results. Aesthetic wax studies and trials are invaluable for patient education and also as a diagnostic aid. Aesthetic study refers to the conventional technique of fabricating wax teeth to simulate the expected result of the definitive restoration.

Duplicate study casts are poured and the abutment teeth prepared approximating to the expected clinical preparations. An aesthetic study in dentine and enamel wax is created. This is invaluable for assessing the likely outcome before any invasive surgery, by using aesthetic wax to assimilate restorations the patient may have a very realistic estimation of the final result. (Roge and Preston, 1987/6)

A clear plastic stent fabricated over a cast of the wax study may be used to aid reduction of the teeth during preparation. (Goldstein, 1970. Gysi, 1982) In addition, it could be used to construct the provisional bridge.

Aesthetic wax trials

Aesthetic wax trials for diagnostic purpose are used to provide an accurate assessment for tissue control, tooth morphology and position. Crown thickness may be measured and feasibility of the recommended procedures verified. In this way it is

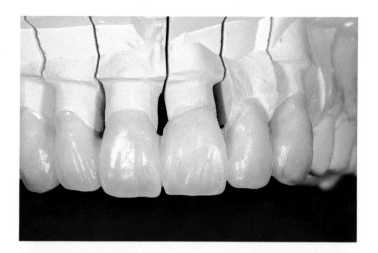

Fig 113 Aesthetic wax trial seen on the working cast provides ceramists with a greater degree of aesthetic possibilities.

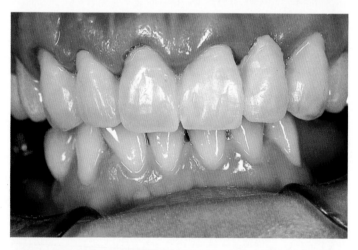

Fig 114 The wax trial is tried in, alterations can be accomplished easily.

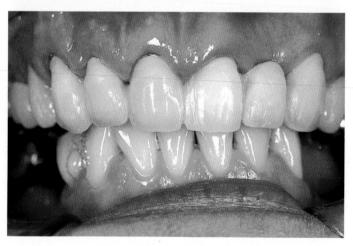

Fig 115 Adjustments were made to the incisal length and the left lateral incisor was reduced at the cervical third. Had these alterations been left until the ceramic stage, quite severe problems would have been encountered, compromising the entire bridge.

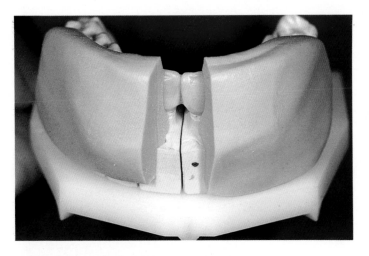

Fig 116 A silicone guide is fabricated over the wax diagnostic trial.

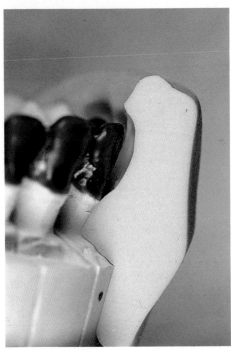

Fig 117 The silicone guide is used to check the wax design for the metal substrate.

possible to create more harmonious aesthetic restorations. The wax restorations are tried in the mouth and alterations are then carried out easily. (Roge, 1988)

The trials are fabricated prior to metal substrate design, however, the technique differs from the usual full contour and cut back in that wax trials are not reduced and subsequently cast to form the metal substrate, but retained and used as a prototype for the definitive work. Silicone indices are fabricated to use as an aid to metal substrate design and ceramic contours (see Chapter 8, page 135)

Waxing directly onto the metal substrate is contraindicated as any alteration in position may invalidate the substrate and in addition, the wax will need to be removed for application of ceramic veneers, thereby losing the aesthetic guide.

After assessment in the mouth, the wax trials are retained and interchanged with the ceramic restoration during its fabrication, to assist contouring.

5.2 Tissue Control with Diagnostic Wax Teeth

Inappropriate tooth contour occurs when the design does not take into account tissue position. Damage is often caused by incorrect emergence profile as under or overcontoured marginal areas cause damage to periodontium. Cases with defficient interdental papillae can lead to unsightly dark spaces between teeth. This is often the result of previous restorative treatment, such as traumatic surgical procedures, poor marginal fit or improperly shaped crown contours. Therefore, crown emergence profile, which is in harmony with periodontal tissue, is essential. Many patients dislike the dark interdental spaces which result when interdental papillae have been lost. Attentive shaping in wax will provide a quick remedy to this.

Not only aesthetics, but also the long-term health of the tissues will result from knowledge of the correct morphologic contour for hygiene and biologic acceptability. Corrections executed as an after-thought to completed crowns and bridges often cause problems for bio-compatibility and aesthetics.

To ascertain correct contour, the wax trial is placed over the prepared teeth. Observations are made to see the effect upon soft tissues and whether the wax restoration is over or under contoured. Tooth anatomy and position are studied for the most

Figs 118 and 119 Soft tissue cast reproduces the position of the gingivae after retraction, causing possible overcontouring of crown margins.

Fig 118

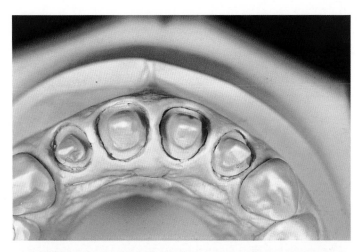

Fig 119

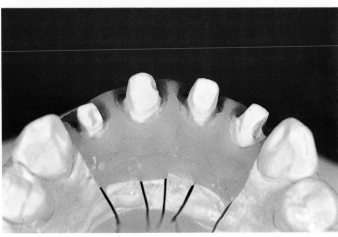

Fig 120 Overcontoured crowns, resulting from the soft tissue model technique which has reproduced the tissue position after gingival retraction, whilst the tissues are still dilated.

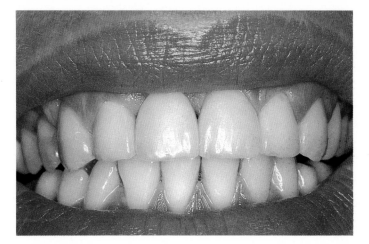

aesthetic result. The wax trial is removed and alterations are carried out. This process is repeated until the desired result is achieved.

An uneven gingival course, especially when comparing one maxillary central to its neighbour, can create aesthetic problems. Diagnostic wax trials are a valuable aid in visualizing tissue contours. Their relationship to the restoration can be verified and if thought necessary, recontoured by the dentist.

Soft Tissue Replication or Wax Trials

The use of Silicone* to replicate the soft tissues as an aid to contour (Kuwata, 1986. Kuwata, 1980) can provide valuable information. However, quite often, impressions will be taken with dilated tissues and so provide an inaccurate representation of the tissue. It follows that restora-made to this information will be over-contoured (fig 120).

5.3 Aesthetic Diagnosis

Where there is a substantial loss of natural dentition, ceramists often feel constrained in their creative ability to replace the missing tooth structures. Variations in tooth position, length, long axes, incisal shape and root formation are all possible for natural effect, however, to create an aesthetic restoration in porcelain requires a heavy investment in time and effort, often the technician is unsure of the design for the restoration and, therefore, the safe option will prevail. This will mean teeth set in regular fashion with very little character, thereby imparting an artificial appearance.

Provisional units can provide useful information for aesthetic harmony, however, unless the wax for the provisional has been tried in the mouth, all the same limiting factors will apply. In addition, the contour of the restoration in the tissue region cannot be transferred to the working cast.

By testing ideas in wax the technician can have the confidence to create natural aesthetics in porcelain.

Wax, by its nature, is not able to withstand biting forces, therefore, patients are instructed not to bite heavily onto the wax trials. Verification of occlusal contact and incisal guidance is also contraindicated for similar reasons.

*Gingifast. Zhermack, 45021 Badia Polesine (Rovigo), Italy.

5.4 Diagnostic Wax Techniques

The fabrication of natural coloured restorations in wax combines the techniques of waxing for metal casting and the artistry of ceramics. Similar principles to ceramic layering are applied to the waxing technique, with the possibility of creating many of the characters present in natural dentition.

Various manufacturers have developed tooth coloured waxes and experience will enable technicians to develop techniques, perhaps utilizing waxes from different sources. Variety exists not only in the subtle colour variations, but also in opacity. It is this quality that can prove to be useful in the aesthetic fabrication.

As in ceramics, coloured waxes are utilized to simulate high chroma dentines, secondary dentine, mamelons, incisal halo, brightened enamel, translucent areas and other characteristics.

An additional benefit would be the use of aesthetic waxes by students to learn the subtleties of colour layering techniques for both ceramics and acrylic restorations.

Techniques for application follow the normal principles for the laying of wax patterns, however, the need to build-in colour requires a layering technique similar to that employed when building ceramics.

Practical application

Understanding where dentine and enamel layers influence the colour in natural dentition will aid the visualization and placement of coloured waxes.

The die is lubricated with a wax release agent.*

Waxes from the 'Belle Art' wax creation set are used.**

High chroma dentine colour is applied using yellow wax, this is placed at the aproximal wall and palatal fossae, if dentine colour is present at the neck or there is the need to form a root, this is also created in yellow wax.

Dentine coloured wax is laid over the preparation to form an internal dentine form. An incisal halo is waxed using blue transparent, care must be exercised to ensure only a fine rim of blue wax is placed. In wax, as in ceramics, excessive use of blue will cause an unnatural appearance.

Enamel, grey translucent and white translucent waxes are used to overlay the dentine and incisal areas to form the enamel overlay, palatal marginal ridges may be formed with white translucent wax for additional character, if required.

Light scattering effects at the incisal edge. The familiar dentine coloured halo surrounding bluish translucency may be simulated with a very thin rim of white translucent wax.

* Microfilm. Kerr (Europe) AG CH-4051 Basel, Switzerland.

** *Yetti Dentalprodukte Gmbh, D.7700 Singen, Postfach 349, Germany.*

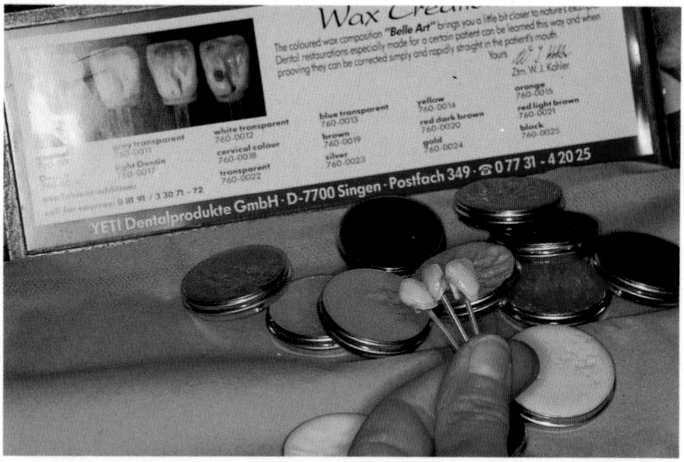

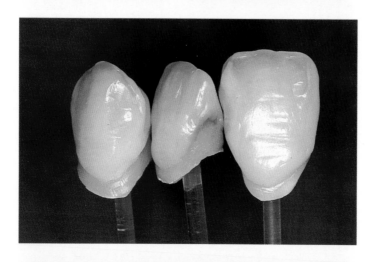

Fig 121 Wax Creation Set from Yeti provides aesthetic possibilities for wax trials.

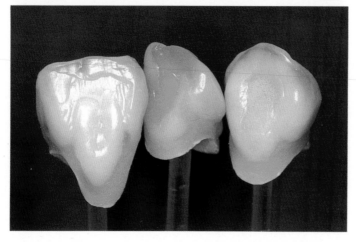

Fig 122 Aesthetic wax teeth demonstrate the many possibilities for creativity.

Fig 123 Palatal aspect.

The wax pattern is carefully trimmed to create both anatomic detail and a natural colour. The avoidance of over waxing will be of benefit at this stage, as excessive trimming of the enamel layer to achieve correct tooth contours will severely compromise the colour. Whilst the possibility of cutting back the dentine layer and re-applying enamel layers may produce the desired result, optimal aesthetics are only attained with correct placement of dentine and enamel layers at the initial waxing stage.

Stages in Laying Aesthetic Waxes

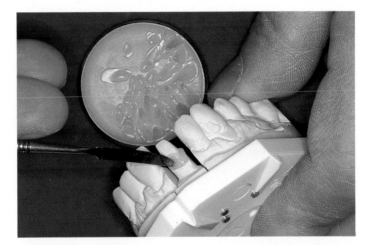

Fig 124 Root dentine colour is simulated by using yellow wax.

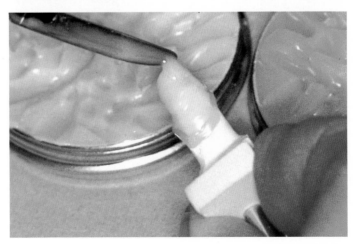

Fig 125 Dentine colour is used to build the dentine core Care must be taken to avoid overcontouring as this will compromise the enamel layer.

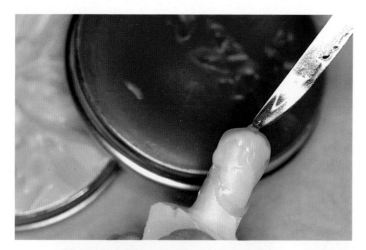

Fig 126 A fine margin of blue wax is laid. This will generate a natural translucent 'halo' effect.

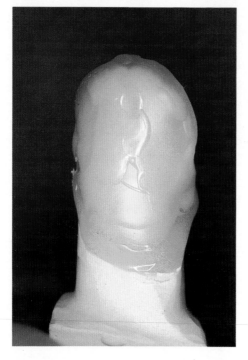

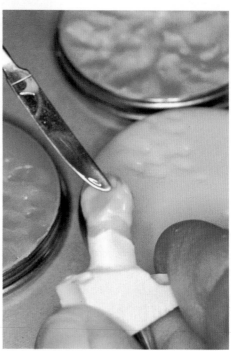

Fig 127 Close detail of wax layers. Yellow root, lighter dentine and blue incisal edge are all clearly evident.

Fig 128 Yellow wax is flowed into the palatal fossae to create high chroma dentine.

Figs 129 to 132 Example of waxing stages for maxillary central incisors with translucent halo and the simulated effect of Raleigh scattering.

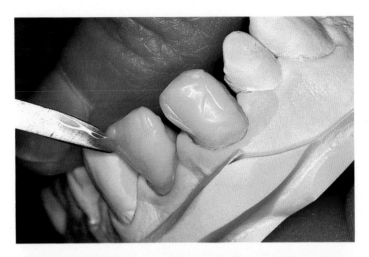

Fig 129 Yellow wax for the root and dentine wax for the body of the tooth are layered.

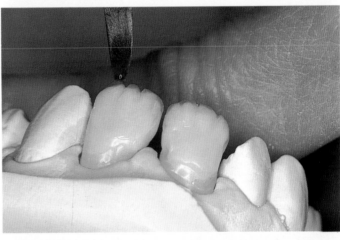

Fig 130 Incisal edge of dentine has been shaped to form dentine mamelons and a fine rim of blue wax is laid to form the translucent halo.

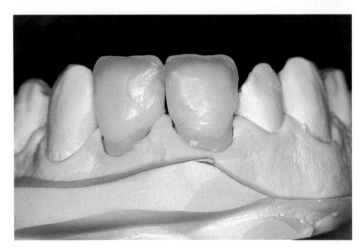

Fig 131 Completed wax crowns, note a fine bead of white translucent wax completes the incisal edge halo.

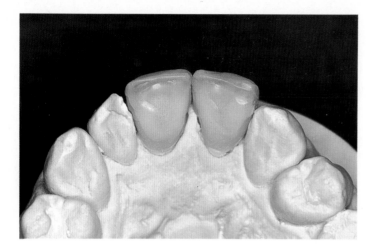

Fig 132   Palatal view.

References

1. *Goldstein R.E:* Esthetics in Dentistry. Ippincott. Philadelphia 1970.
2. *Gysi B.E:* in Esthetic Guidelines for Restorative Dentistry pp 105 Quintessence Pub. Co. Inc. Chicago, Illinois 1982.
3. *Kuwata M:* Ceramo-Metal Technology Vol 1. pp 72-79 Ishmaku Euro America Inc. St Louis. 1986.
4. *Kuwata M:* Theory and Practice for Ceramo-Metal Restorations pp 78-81 Quintessence Pub. Co. Inc. Chicago, Illinois 1980.
5. *Roge M. & Preston J. D:* Color, Light and the Perception of Form: Quintessence International 1987/6.
6. *Roge M:* Evaluation and Control in Aesthetic Dentistry. 7th Quintessence International Symposium. Paris 1988.

6 Accurate Registration and Communication of Colour Characteristics

From our observation of natural dentition, it is clear there are many subtle colour characteristics within the tooth structure. The problem is how to record information in such a way as to be able to produce exactly what we have seen in dental porcelain.

This chapter provides techniques which will enable the dentist and technician to reproduce colour characteristics with more accuracy and realism.

6.1 Commercial Colour System

To create a tooth that is truly able to match its counterpart in the oral environment, it is essential the technician has a range of colours that allow a close match to the characteristic required.

Most current porcelain systems have developed specialized frits to match many of the colour characteristics seen in natural dentition.

The Ivoclar Porcelain System (IPS) contains the Paul Muir (1982) Maverick System, mamelon colours, coloured translucent frits for reproducing incisal halo effects, a special frit of the whiter enamel seen on the occlusal of posterior teeth and a range of opalescent enamels. In addition, many frits such as opacious dentine and intensive dentines enable technicians to build lifelike restorations.

The Duceram Creative Color System (Hegenbath E. 1989) uses nature's example and contains 26 colours associated with the internal characteristics of human dentition, these include incisal mamelon, secondary dentine, root shades and a range of incisal blue colours.

Commercial shade guides have only limited success in achieving accurate shade analysis. Apart from the obvious differences between the commercial guide and a metal-ceramic crown such as differing thickness and

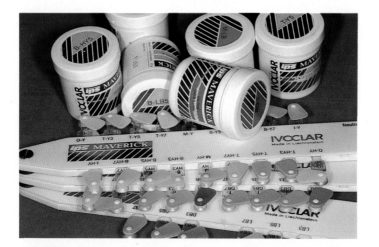

Figs 133 and 134 Ivoclar Maverick and Impulse shade selectors provide the technician with many possibilities for building characteristics.

Fig 133

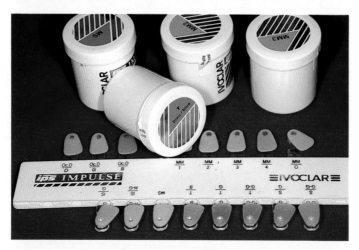

Fig 134

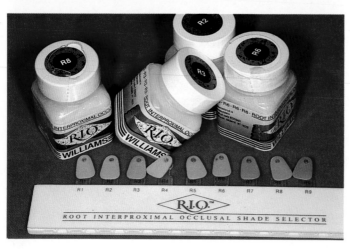

Fig 135 Ivoclar/Williams have formulated a range of high chroma dentines to simulate dentine in the root, interproximal and occlusal areas.

Figs 136 and 137 Original Doric Root Shades* and the new R.I.O. tabs.

* Davis Schottlander & Davis Ltd. Brimsley Centre, Dunhams Lane, Letchworth, Herts, England.

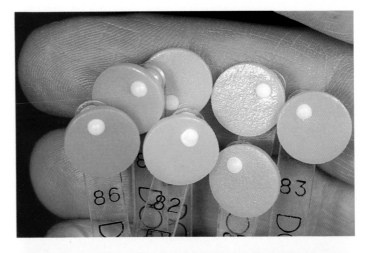

Fig 136

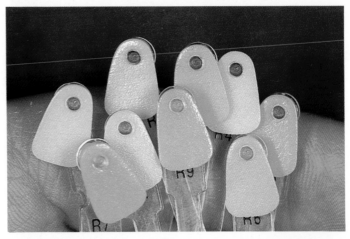

Fig 137

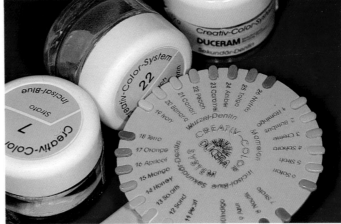

Fig 138 Duceram Creative Color Wheel contains 26 shades for building colour characteristics.

structure, it is clearly evident that a crown with only 1mm of porcelain veneer, including a highly reflective opaque layer, has very little chance of matching the commercial shade guides. Ducera have introduced their Duceram-on-Metal Selector, however, this has limitations as it bears little resemblance to the aesthetic possibilities which many dental technicians are able to achieve.

The natural progression is for the technician to fabricate his own individual shade guide. This guide is described as the Characteristic Shade Guide.

6.2 The Characteristic Shade Guide

The characteristic shade guide utilizes the Vita* individual guide and is custom fabricated to include the characteristics of mamelon, incisal blue, root/high chroma dentine and enamel brightening. The advantages of this guide are that it provides a physical simulation of how the colour characteristics are seen with the technician's own technique. The guide is fabricated from ceramic materials normally used and built by the technician, thereby reproducing a shade guide system pertinent to the individual technician. (Buzola FN. 1967)

* Vita Zahnfabrik, D-7880 Bad Sackingen, Postfach 1338. Germany.

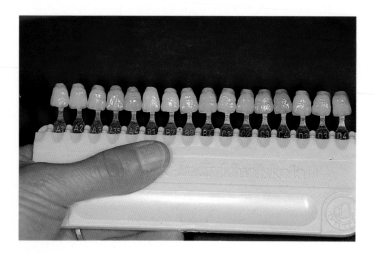

Fig 139 The characteristic guide is fabricated using the Vita Individual guide.

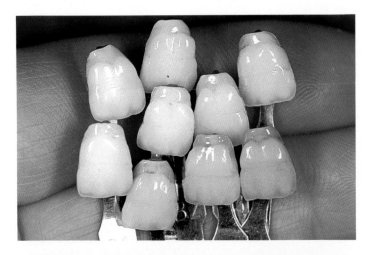

Fig 140 Selection of shades from the characteristic guide.

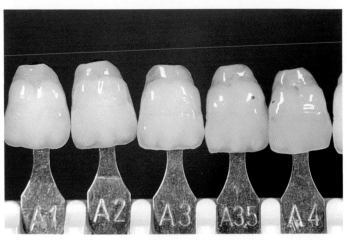

Fig 141 Close detail of the 'A' range.

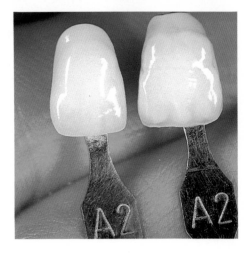

Fig 142 Close detail depicting shade Vita A2.

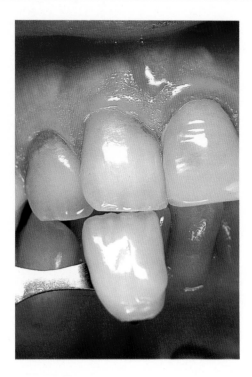

Fig 143 Characteristic guide in use. As in many instances the guide is very close to the natural characteristics seen in the mouth.

Custom Shade Tabs

There are times when the custom shade guide does not match and guessing at blends of ceramic hues is often inadequate. The only recourse for a predictable result is for the technician to fabricate a custom shade tab in the laboratory. This takes a little time but is well worth the effort, often saving many remakes.

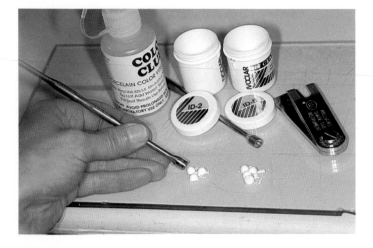

Figs 144 to 150 Demonstrate the technique employed to build a custom shade tab of a difficult maxillary central, after several attempts to fabricate a satisfactory crown.

Fig 144 Ceramic colours are measured with volumetric scoops.

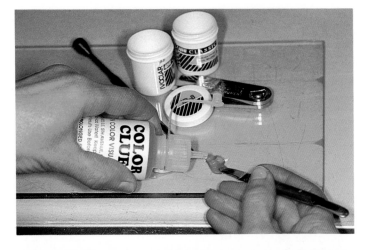

Fig 145 Color Clue Liquid is used to visualize the correct colour. Additional ceramic colours are added until the correct combination is achieved. Careful notes are kept to record the mixture.

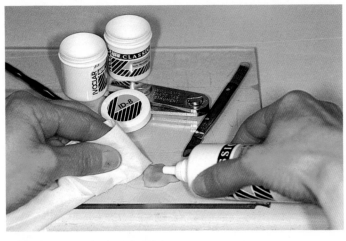

Fig 146 Color Clue Liquid needs to be removed from the porcelain to facilitate the building of a large mass. Modelling liquid is used to saturate the mixture and tissue is employed to soak up excess liquid, eventually all the Color Clue Liquid is removed.

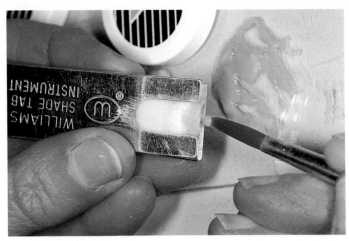

Fig 147 The custom shade tab is built. In this example a white band is laid in the body area and a translucent blue/grey mixture at the incisal third.

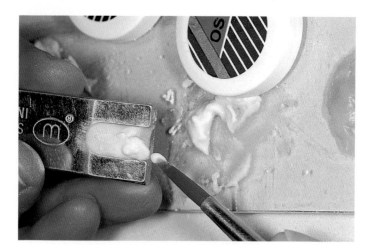

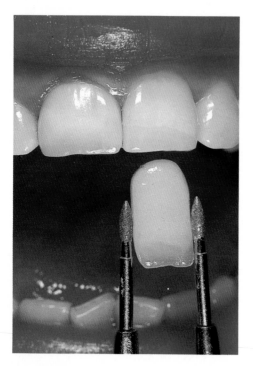

Fig 148 Enamel porcelain is overlaid.

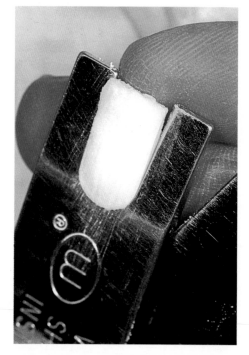

Fig 149 The Williams tab maker opens in a scissor-like fashion, enabling the tab to be removed for sintering.

Fig 150 After several attempts a successful colour tab is fabricated, matching the natural right central. Left central is the previous poor match.

6.3 Enamel-Dentine Distribution

We have all experienced the dilemma when a restoration appears to match the shade guide, yet is a poor match when placed in the mouth. One of the predominating causes for this phenomenon is due to a mismatch in the enamel-dentine distribution. Layering techniques in ceramics are capable of varying the depth of enamel overlay, as well as the extent of enamel influence towards the cervical third. The degree of translucency or opacity has a direct bearing on the value of the shade. With such variables it is important to record any variance from the normal distribution seen on the shade guide, and to be aware of the value, translucency and distribution of the enamel layer.

The appearance and effect of the enamel overlay may be difficult for a dental surgeon to communicate to the technician. However, some attempt should be made to provide information with regard to the extent of the enamel overlay towards the tooth cervix and the depth of translucency or degree of opacity.

Technicians fortunate enough to be able to see first hand during shade selection procedures should sketch the enamel-dentine distribution and make written notes of exact building technique. It is only by making a detailed assessment of the layering technique to be employed, with the patient in attendance, that some success may be accomplished. For difficult cases a shade tab should be fired whilst the patient waits. Of course careful notation of mixtures and layering technique is mandatory.

6.4 Communication Through Photography

Photographic equipment has advanced to the point where it is possible for both the dentist and technician to achieve high quality photographs capable of communicating information, with respect to a number of dental applications. The use of photographs to convey the characteristics of colour in natural dentition is a prime example. By placing the guide in the photograph it is possible to transfer the information to the technician.

Whilst photographic technology is not sufficiently sophisticated to transmit the exact shade, it is possible to convey the value of teeth in relation to the shade guide (fig 151). The individual characteristics such as mamelon, crack lines, root shades or unusual shades can also be recorded on film. The use of a colour corrected light box or slide viewer will prevent colour distortion of the photograph.

The aesthetic appearance of restorations at bisque trial or indeed any prosthetic appliance is another of the many uses for dental photography.

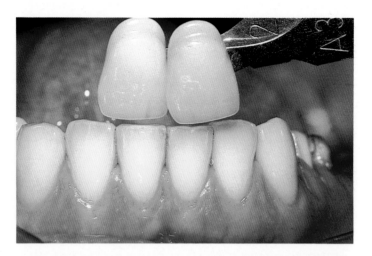

Fig 151 Placing the shade guide in the photograph provides information on the relative colour aspects to the natural situation. In this case the natural teeth exhibit a high value compared to the guide.

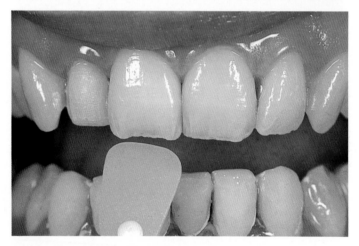

Figs 152 and 153 Communication through a photograph of the many colour characteristics provides a clear understanding of precise colour and distribution.

Fig 152

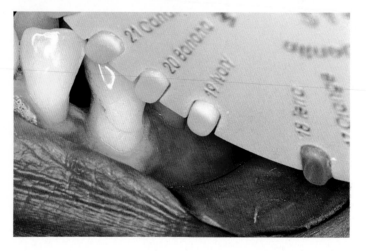

Fig 153

Slide transparencies are preferred to colour prints as colour reproduction is more reliable. In particular, the superior reproduction of transparent and translucent areas within the incisal region. The least predictable are Polaroid photographs which have a tendency to alter in colour balance.

Disadvantages of slide transparencies are that the shortest film run is 24 exposures. This can cause a problem of delay in waiting for the complete film to be used. The only effective way around this is to ignore the cost and process a partly exposed film. It is possible to go into a dark room and open the camera to withdraw the exposed section, cut-off and process, however, the cost of processing will be the same for a part film as for a complete run so little advantage is gained.

Colour prints are preferred when making a practice case book to enable patients to visualize differing forms of treatment, for this purpose high quality prints provide the ideal solution.

Equipment

There are a number of manufacturers able to supply excellent photographic equipment. It is important that the system is able to correctly expose with an aperture of F16 or smaller. Apertures larger than this will cause loss of depth of field, that is, central incisors will be in focus but canines will not.

Twin flash units are preferable to a ring flash as the latter tends to create a high degree of surface reflection with a circular highlight in the centre of the tooth, this is not so critical on natural dentition but has the effect of exposing every blemish on ceramic veneers.

The use of a dedicated flash unit with through-the-lens metering of the exposure will save a lot of trial and error and the need to bracket shots.

Macro camera equipment used routinely in the author's laboratory and for intra-oral photography comprises:

Camera Body	Olympus 101
Lens	Vivitar 105mm Macro
2 × Converter	D01 HQ7
Flash Unit	Olympus T 28 twin flash fitted with opal diffuser. Olympus Ring Flash
Film	Kodak Ektachrome Professional 100 and 200

References

1. *Buzola F. N.* & *Molone W. F:* Shade Guide for Vacuum-Fired-Porcelain-Gold Crowns. S. American Dental Association 74:114 1967.
2. *Hegenbath E:* Creating Ceramic Colour: A Practical System. Quintessence Publishing Co. Inc. Chicago, Illinois. USA 1989.
3. *Muia P. J:* Four Dimensional Tooth Color System. Quintessence Publishing Co. Inc. 1982. Chicago

7 Advanced Laboratory Techniques

7.1 Methods for an Aesthetic Ceramic Margin (Metal Ceramics)

The concept of shoulder preparations for ceramic margins has been advocated for improved aesthetics for many years, as long ago as 1977 Toogood and Archibald pioneered the research into ways of achieving all ceramic margins. Since those early days many styles have evolved. Three approaches achieved wide acceptance viz methods using platinum foil, lift off techniques with wax and ceramic mixtures and the direct lift off technique.

Initially, metal subframes were only slightly reduced at the labial margin. Problems existed due to insufficient space and a shadow cast from the metal substrate causing the tooth root to appear grey. It was for this reason that techniques were devised to substantially reduce the metal substrate, with each advance advocating further reduction of the metal.

Vryonis (1979) developed improved techniques by a larger reduction at the shoulder and extending the reduction up the axial wall by 0.4mm. Geller (1990) has developed the concept further, by advocating reduction of the axial wall by up to 4mm.

Technique for the aesthetic ceramic margin

The following examples describe variations of the direct lift off technique using conventional margin porcelains.

Different layering techniques for the construction of the ceramic margin will depend upon the amount of tooth reduction and also the reduction of the metal substrate. A further consideration will be whether optimal aesthetics is required. Often margins which are not visible, that is, in the posterior region or lower incisors, do not require such a high degree of aesthetics and Type A or B margin technique may be adequate. Where optimal aesthetics at the margin are required, precise preparation with a shoulder width of 1.5mm is necessary (fig 157, Type D).

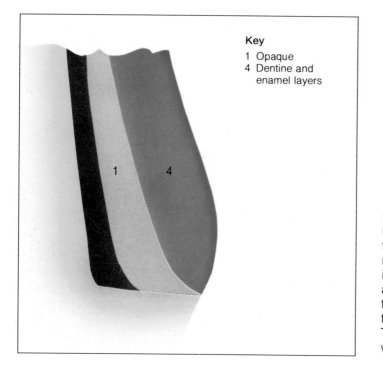

Key
1 Opaque
4 Dentine and
   enamel layers

Fig 154   Type A
Minimal reduction of the metal to allow 0.3mm for ceramic margin, in this example there is insufficient room for opaque and margin porcelain and for this reason the opaque is taken to the full extent of the margin. This technique is ideal for cases with limited shoulder width.

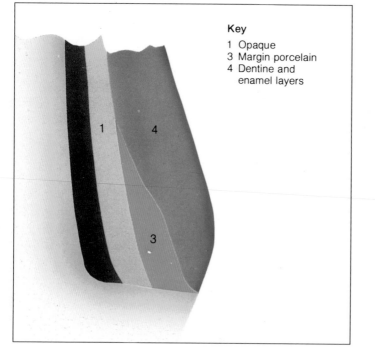

Key
1 Opaque
3 Margin porcelain
4 Dentine and
   enamel layers

Fig 155   Type B
Maximum reduction of the metal substrate across the width of the shoulder allows the use of margin porcelains. Providing a greater depth for overlays reduces the high value and reflective nature of the opaque. However, both Type A and B do not allow light to penetrate through the crown margin, therefore, shadows from the metal substrate will still adversely affect the colour of the tooth root.

Fig 156   Type C
A further advance in the design for the aesthetic margin was developed by Vryonis (1979), who recognised the importance of allowing light to enter the tooth root. By reducing the metal to a maximum of 0.4 mm in a coronal direction, improved results were evident.

However, it was found necessary to apply opaque to the apical margin of the metal to avoid metallic shadows transmitting through the margin porcelain. This left very little depth for margin material (0.2 mm) and whilst an improvement over Type B was achieved it was of minimal value, as the space available for light transmission to the tooth root was insufficient to achieve optimal results.

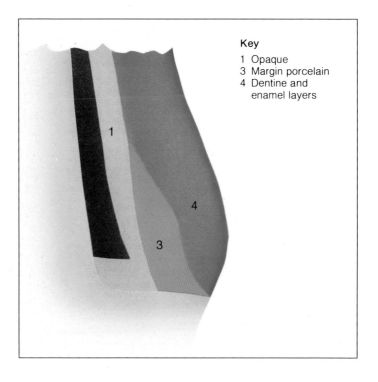

Key
1 Opaque
3 Margin porcelain
4 Dentine and
    enamel layers

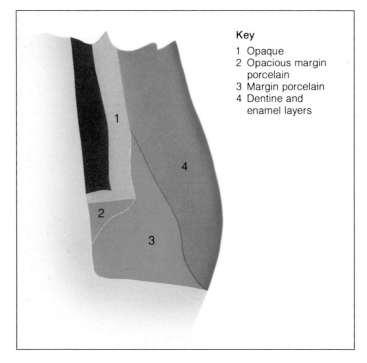

Key
1 Opaque
2 Opacious margin
    porcelain
3 Margin porcelain
4 Dentine and
    enamel layers

Fig 157   Type D
Reduction of the metal substrate by as much as 4 mm has been advocated by Geller. The reason for this is quite clear as the problem of grey shadows in the root area had still not been fully overcome.

This technique represents the fullest extent by which a metal substrate can be reduced. Allowing maximum light penetration of the tooth root through the margin porcelain. The technique is very time consuming as up to four or five margin firings are necessary to achieve optimum results, often the shoulder porcelain will distort away from the preparation and additions to compensate are necessary. Undercut areas must be eliminated, as even a small one will prevent a successful lift off and cause breakage of the green porcelain.

Comparison of light transmission through the porcelain margin with increasing degrees of metal substrate reduction.

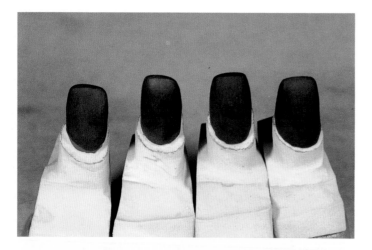

Fig 158 Oxidized metal on dies.

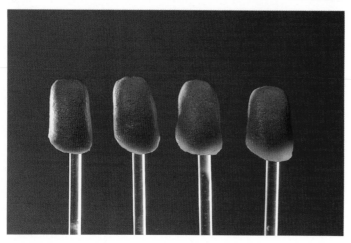

Fig 159 Light transmitted through the margin.

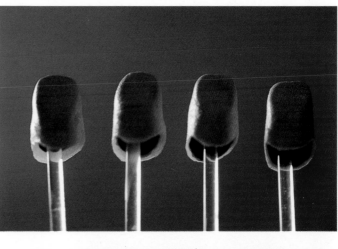

Fig 160   Palatal view.

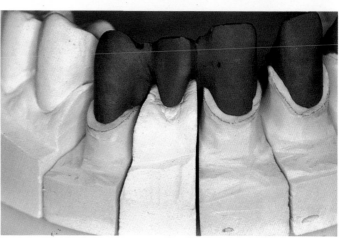

Fig 161   Bridge case demonstrates maximum reduction across shoulder. Note the provision of a good shoulder width of 1.5mm to allow depth of porcelain. This is essential to mask reflective opaque layers. Three firings of margin porcelain are normally required to achieve a close marginal fit.

Duplicate dies in epoxy resin*

Many technicians have problems with the direct lift off method, and a variety of techniques and materials have been advocated to improve this. Developments such as light curing liquids or the use of colloidial silica to bind the ceramic into a solid state prior to lift off have been advocated.

The use of duplicate epoxy resin dies has proved to be beneficial as it is ideal for the clean separation of porcelain margin material. The use of die sealant is not necessary, as the material does not absorb moisture.

* Epoxy Die. Ivoclar, Schaan, Leichtenstein.

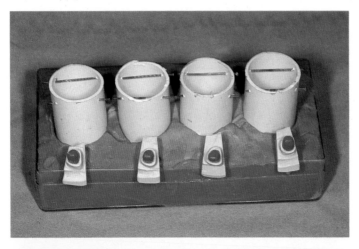

Fig 162 Plastic pipe is sectioned and used as duplicating rings. Steel dressmaker's pins are heated and inserted into the ring to support the stone die.

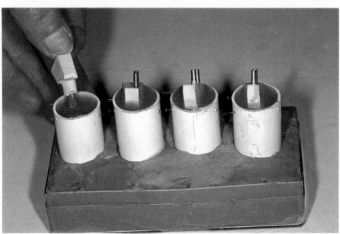

Fig 163 Silicone Duplicating Material** is vacuum stirred to form an air free mixture and poured into the ring. The stone die is carefully positioned.

** Elite Double. Zhermack, 45021 Badia Polesine (Rovigo) Italy.

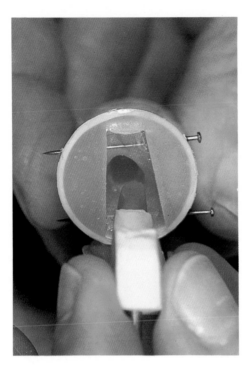
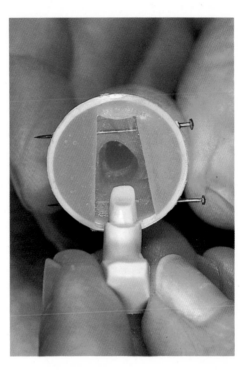

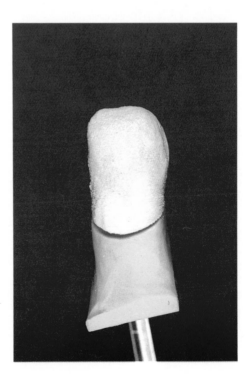

Fig 164 When the silicone material has set the die is removed and epoxy material is mixed and cast into the duplicate mould.

Fig 165 Removal of the epoxy resin die.

Fig 166 Epoxy resin is ideal for ceramic lift off techniques, facilitating a clean separation without the use of die sealant.

7.2 Opalescence

Opalescence is the term given to substances which exhibit similar properties to opal stone when subjected to transmitted or reflected light. Viewed under normal conditions, that is, in reflected light, an opal has a blue appearance as most of the short wavelength is reflected. However, when transilluminated, an opal will appear amber, this is due to the light scattering properties of the stone splitting and filtering the light beam, allowing only the longer (0.59-0.7μm) wavelength component to be transmitted through the opal. These longer wavelengths are those in the red/orange range of the light spectrum, hence the orange tint when transilluminated. This phenomenon is also found in natural dentition within the enamel layer due to the hydroxyapatite crystal and other structures diffusing and scattering the light beam. (Yamamoto, 1985)

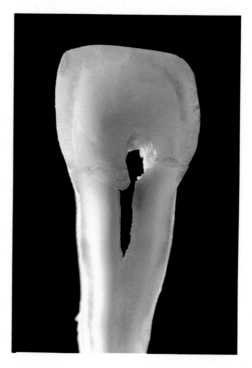

Fig 167 Natural tooth mesiodistal longitudinal ground section. Transillumination reveals opalescent qualities. See also figs 51 and 52, Chapter 1.2.

Opalescence in dental ceramic

True opalescence is caused by the inclusion of sub-wavelength particles (300 nanometers) within the ceramic frit. These fine particles need to be smaller than the light beam, splitting the light and causing the short wave length to scatter, it is this that gives the opalescent quality.

NB. All samples are photographed using a Phillips tungsten Reflecta bulb and Kodak Ektachrome tungsten film.

Figs 168 to 170 Demonstrate the opalescence of Ivoclar OS Enamels,* after five firings.

* Ivoclar. Schann, Leichtenstein.

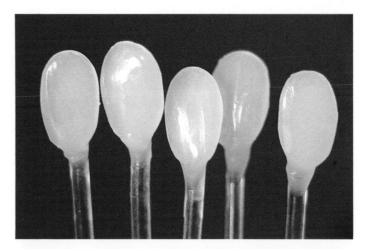

Fig 168 Photographed with reflected light.

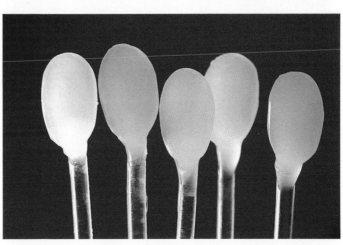

Fig 169 The light source is positioned at the side.

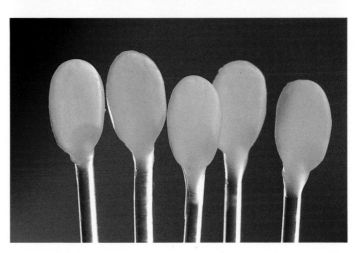

Fig 170 Transilluminated.

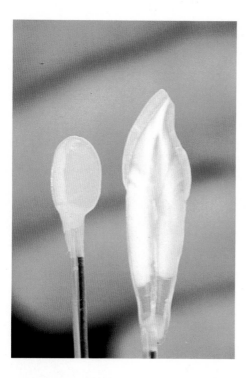

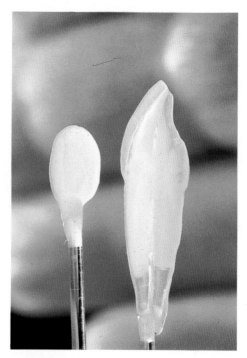

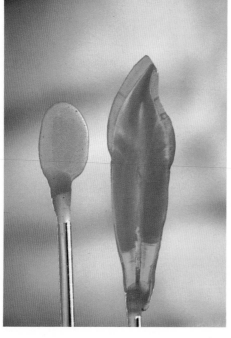

Fig 171 to 173 Opalescent enamels placed within the photograph demonstrate the way they and natural tooth sections react to a rotating light source.

Fig 171 Photographed in reflected light.

Fig 172 The light source is positioned at the side.

Fig 173 Transilluminated.

Figs 174 to 177 Demonstrate the opalescence of 'Duceram LFC Opal', after five firings.

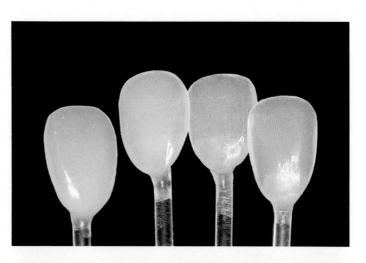

Fig 174 Two tabs on the left are Duceram LFC Opalescent Porcelain, the remaining tabs are Duceram, regular enamel.

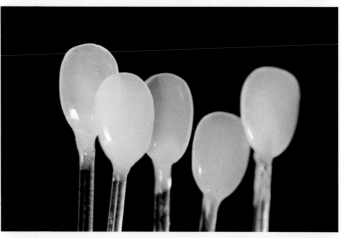

Fig 175 Photographed in reflected light.

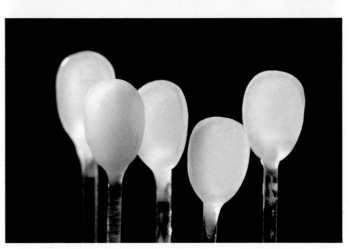

Fig 176 The light source is positioned at the side.

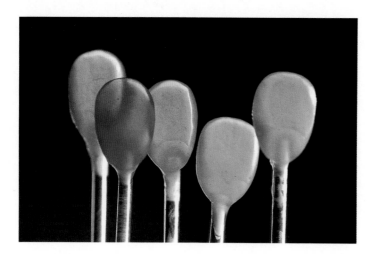

Fig 177   Transilluminated.

7.3 Development of the Dentine Mamelon

One of the most difficult building techniques in ceramics is the formation of dentine mamelons that are typical in the young dentition.

Mamelon structures are the result of lobes emanating from the dentine during the developmental stage, initially they delineate the incisal edge, but are usually worn flat during the early stages of wear (McLean, 1980). It is not unusual for these finger-like structures to become visible through the outer mantle of enamel.

Care must be taken to avoid a pedestrian appearance of regimented lobe formation. Close attention to the shaping of the dentine build-up will provide the key to this elusive characteristic. The finger-like mamelons should be clearly delineated, both at the incisal edge and within the facial aspect of the dentine build-up, thereby creating a three-dimensional appearance.

The mamelon formation may take a variety of forms with three, four or more fingers, as in maxillary central incisors. Where less room cramps the successful formation, as in maxillary lateral incisors or mandibular incisors, a simplified form comprising two fingers may be developed.

It is common for the mamelon form to be incomplete, with the result that it appears feathered or as spots of dentine colour within the enamel structure.

Technique using two sintering stages

First stage: Dentine and mamelon characteristics

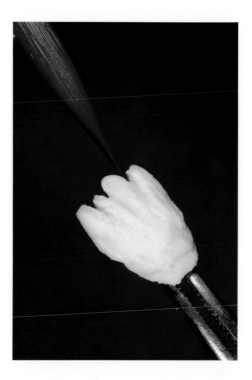

Fig 178 First stage:
Example of dentine cut-back, demonstrating the mamelon formation which extends into the facial anatomy.

Fig 179 A blue modifier is used with Color Clue Liquid (Visual Building Technique) to establish the internal dentine mamelon structure.

Fig 180 The mamelon structures are clearly seen.

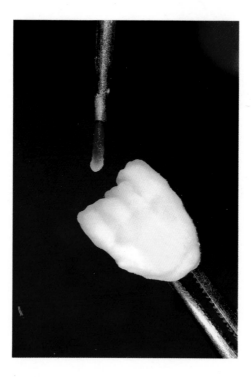

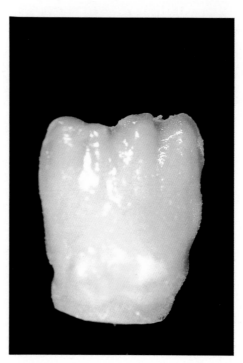

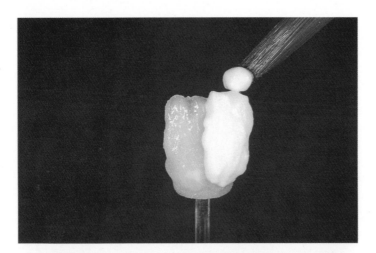

Fig 181 Second stage:
Enamel porcelain layers are built. Due to the pre-fired mamelon and halo characteristics merging of colours is prevented.

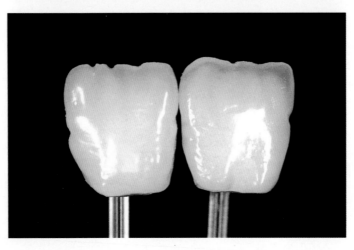

Fig 182 Two examples of mamelon structure with differing cut-back technique.

Second stage: Translucent clear halo effects and enamel layers are built.

The Visual Building Technique is used to build mamelon colour and blue effects to accentuate the mamelon structures. These are carefully placed around each finger or mamelon structure. When mamelon characteristics are complete the build-up is ready for the first dentine firing.

Sintering the build-up at this juncture will provide an opportunity to adjust the level of incisal mamelon structures before continuing to build the transparent halo and enamel layers.

Enamel layers are built using enamel of varying translucency. The incisal halo is completed with a pale dentine effect.

Three stage sintering techniques

Stage one is dentine build-up. In **Stage two** the mamelon characteristics are built after adjusting position and incisal length.
In **Stage three** translucent clear various enamel layers and incisal rim are built.

Fig 183 Following the first stage of building the dentine, adjustments are made to the mamelon structures.

Fig 184 Dentine with mamelon structures.

Fig 185 Second stage:
A blue modifier is placed to increase translucency and sintered.

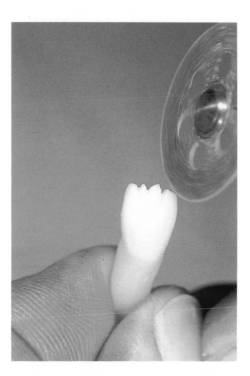

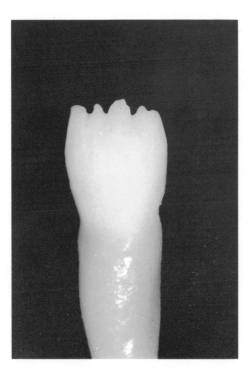

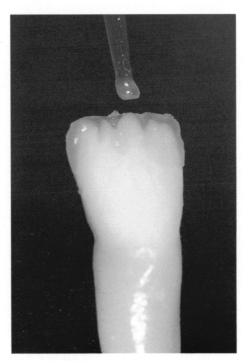

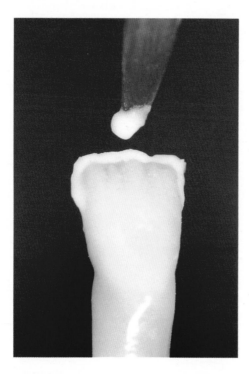

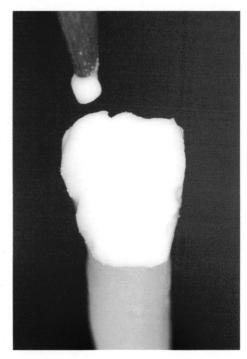

Fig 186 Translucent clear is placed around the dentine and blue modifier.

Fig 187 Third stage: Enamel and incisal rim layers are completed and sintered.

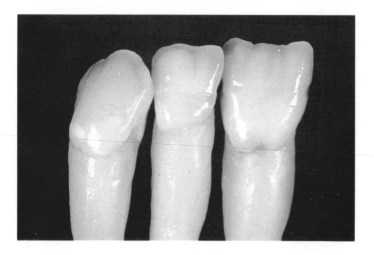

Fig 188 Maxillary teeth for young dentition.

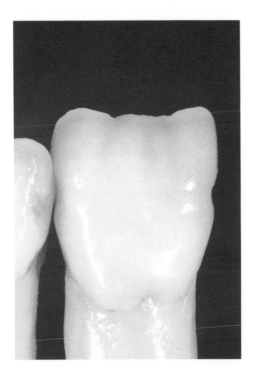

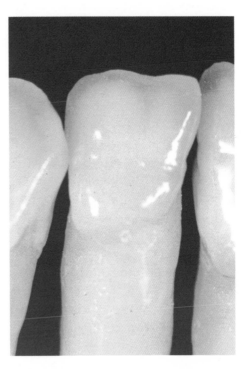

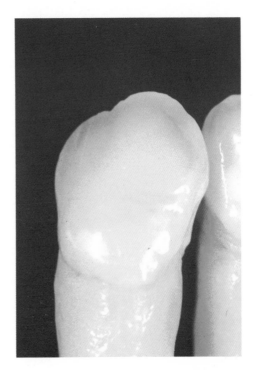

Fig 189   Close detail maxillary central incisor.

Fig 190   Close detail maxillary lateral incisor.

Fig 191   Close detail maxillary canine.

7.4 Aged Dentition using a Multiple Sintering Technique

Complex colour structures such as those found in the middle aged and aged dentition sometimes require multiple sintering techniques. This is because of the multiplicity of such characteristics as crack lines, discoloured spots or pits, wear facets and abrasion characteristics. These characteristics are extremely difficult for even the most competent technician to build with a single bake technique.

At the first stage the dentine structures, including underlying high chroma dentines or opacious dentines, are built. Those characteristics which the technician feels can be executed with success and which lie within the dentine are included at this stage. Enamel translucent and clear zones will be built at a later stage.

After sintering, the dentine structure is adjusted by grinding, fine crack lines may be depicted in the surface. Surface stains are used to characterize the structure and fused in place. Reducing the sintering temperature by approximately 100°C is sufficient to fix these characteristics.

Following this any further characterizations, such as a translucent halo, are built and sintered. Finally, the enamel structures are built.

These techniques enable technicians to build complex structures, with a more predictable result.

Multiple sintering technique for complex colour structures

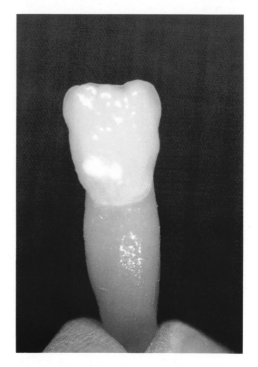

Fig 192 Initial dentine structure with some characteristics in place.

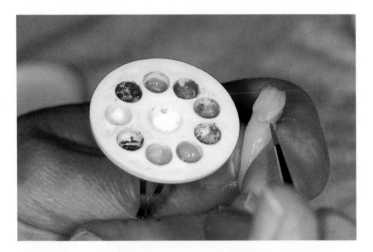

Fig 193 Surface stains are used to further characterize the dentine.

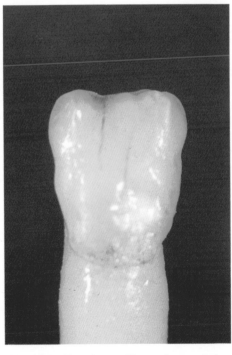

Fig 194 Dentine with surface stains fused in position.

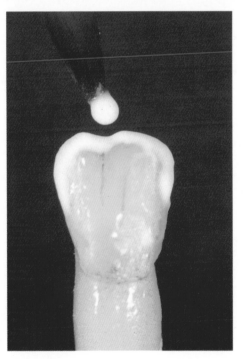

Fig 195 Clear porcelain is used to create a halo effect.

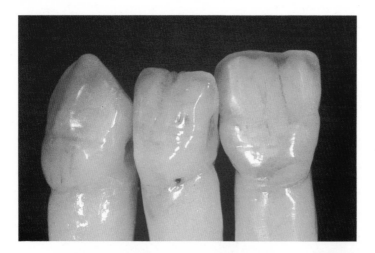

Fig 196 Phantom teeth depict the complex internal colour structures possible with this technique.

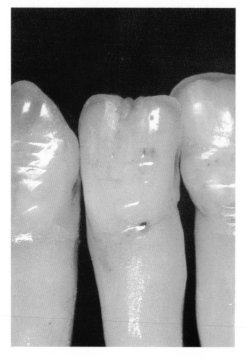

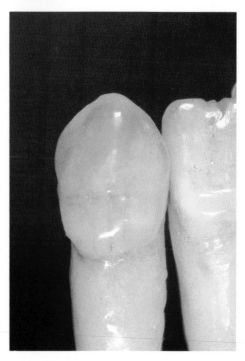

Fig 197 Close detail lateral incisor.

Fig 198 Close detail of the canine.

Figs 199 to 204 Examples of maxillary incisors for the aged dentition demonstrate the use of the multiple sintering technique where complex enamel structures are required.

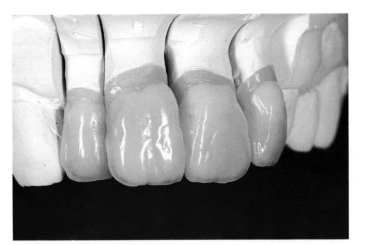

Fig 199 Diagnostic wax crowns aid aesthetic position and form.

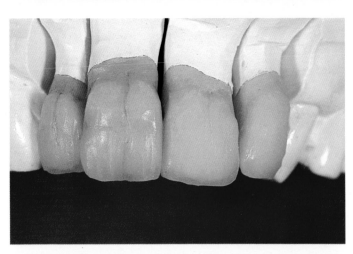

Fig 200 Left central and lateral incisors after stains have been fused to position.

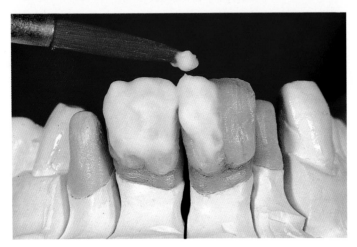

Fig 201 Addition of enamel porcelain over the stained labial surfaces.

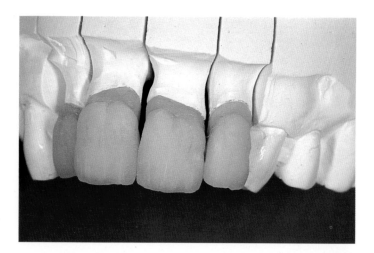

Fig 202 Crowns, after final grinding adjustments, are ready for glazing.

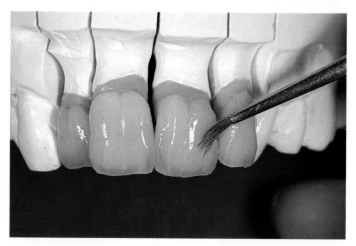

Fig 203 The application of stain fluid shows clearly the internal stained characteristics.

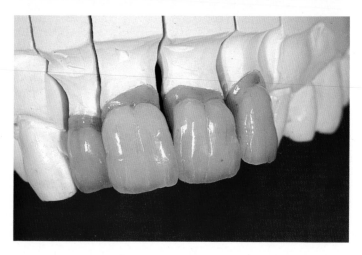

Fig 204 Glazed and polished crowns.

7.5 Anterior Tooth Position and Form

Aesthetic replacement of anterior teeth is as much a question of contour and position as colour. When the restoration is limited to one or two teeth it is not difficult for a competent technician to create natural restorations. Cases requiring four or more anterior teeth become a problem as the visualizing of natural harmony is difficult. The situation is exacerbated by patients' and their dentists' requests for an even arrangement of teeth, as this will very often lead to an unnatural appearance.

Typo-dent study cast

a) Study casts of attractive anterior teeth may be utilized. By collecting casts a selection is available from which the technician will be able to choose an arrangement of natural dentition which has harmony with the case to be restored. This will provide many aesthetic possibilities for tooth position, contour and natural character and will be the source of much inspiration.

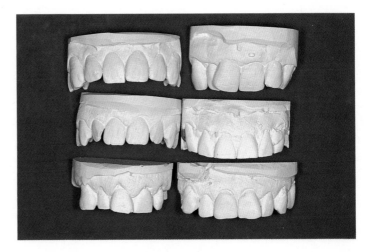

Fig 205 A collection of typo-dent study casts of natural anteriors used for reference to tooth position, contour and character.

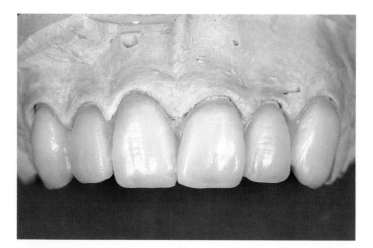

Figs 206 to 208 Wax studies upon the same case demonstrate the unending variety of tooth form and position. Technicians have difficulty imagining such variety, resulting in an unattractive denture-like appearance.

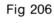

Fig 206

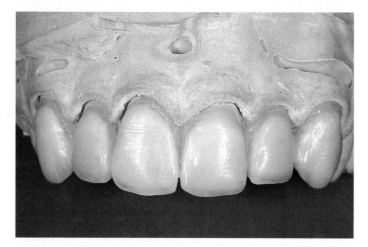

Fig 207

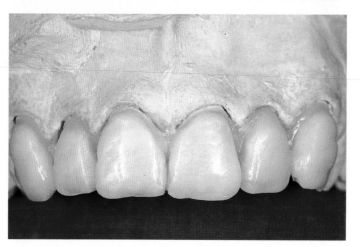

Fig 208

Figs 209 and 210 Wax studies have utilized the Typodent study cast system, giving rise to many varied tooth arrangements.

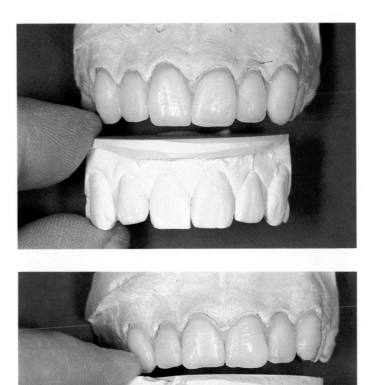

Fig 209

Fig 210

Green articulating spray as an aid to visualizing anatomy

Often, it is the experience of technicians when viewing a cast of a recently fitted restoration that the result is far from satisfactory, the restoration appears obviously different from the natural dentition.

Past techniques have simulated this situation prior to completion of the work, by taking an impression of the ceramic work on the working cast and casting in dental stone. The result provides information, as if the restoration were fitted in the mouth.

The reason that faults are more conspicuous on the cast is due to the dental stone material being a dense, opaque substance. This provides a clearer idea of surface texture and anatomy than semi-translucent

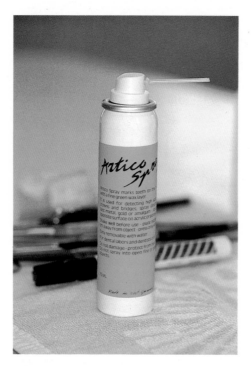

Fig 211 Green articulating spray.

ceramic. If both restoration and natural dentition appear on the cast as a solid substance, that is, as dental stone, the differences between the restoration and remaining natural dentition will be more apparent.

The use of green articulating spray alleviates the need to use such time-consuming procedures. The spray renders the ceramic and stone teeth on the cast as a light green opaque colour, giving a similar appearance to dental stone when assessing tooth anatomy and surface texture.

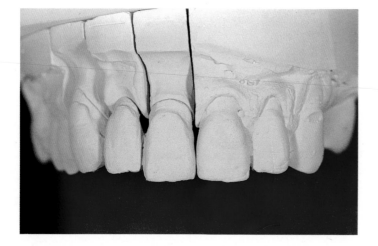

Figs 212 to 214 Examples of three metal/ceramic bridges. Green articulating spray highlights anatomic faults and poor surface texture.

Fig 212 In this example the distal line angle of the right lateral incisor is clearly incorrect and should be angled to give the tooth a more tapered appearance.

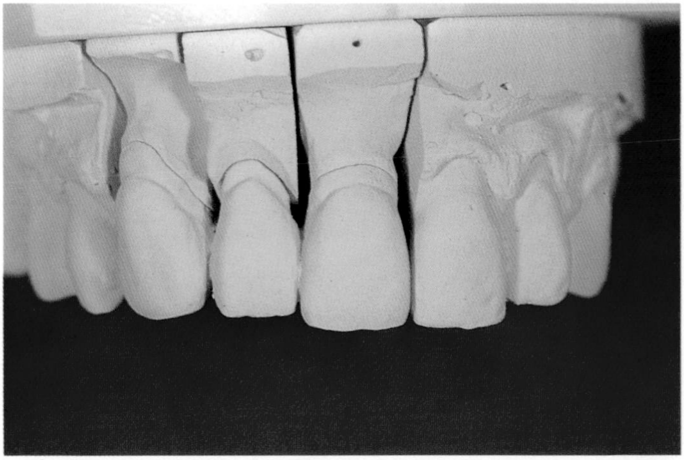

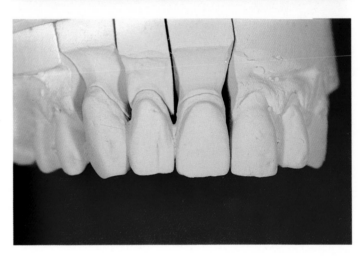

Fig 213 The right central and lateral incisors both appear oversized. The central incisor is too wide and the line angles are rounded.

Fig 214 The right lateral incisor appears too long.

7.6 Study of Posterior Teeth

Technicians need to study actual teeth, rather than plaster casts on which cases are fabricated. These often lack sufficient detail to be of use due to the presence of previous restorations. Studies of natural dentition may be accomplished by acquiring extracted teeth and by the observation of natural dentition *in situ.*

Resin replicas may be purchased and are a useful learning aid, however, these are a poor substitute for the real thing.

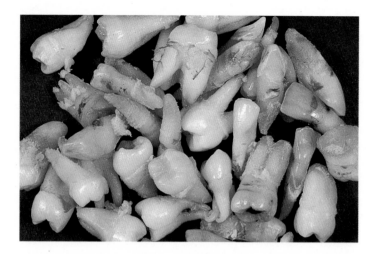

Fig 215 A collection of extracted natural teeth is invaluable for the study of anatomy, structure and character.

Figs 216 to 222 A silicone mould is poured to duplicate the natural teeth.

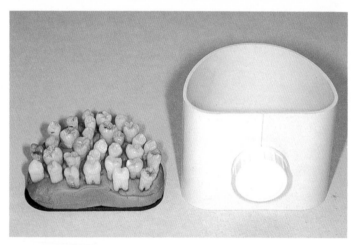

Fig 216 Teeth are embedded into silicone putty material.

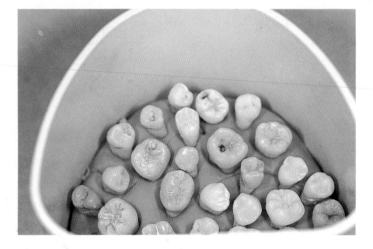

Fig 217 Teeth are placed in the duplicating flask.

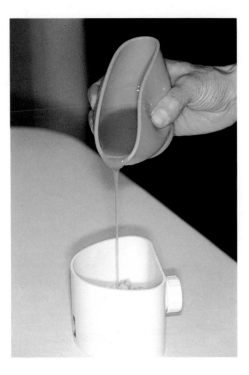

Fig 218 Silicone is poured after vacuum mixing.

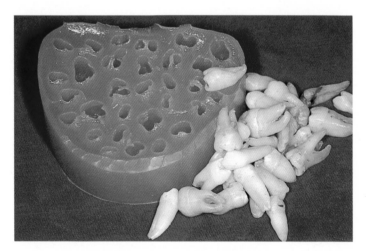

Fig 219 Completed mould ready for casting in dental stone.

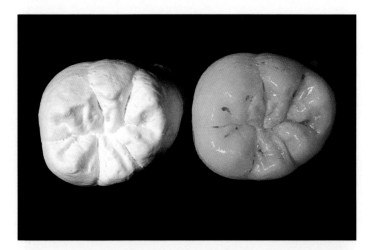

Fig 220 Natural mandibular molar and stone replica.

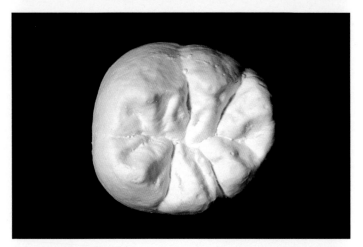

Fig 221 Stone replica clearly details surface anatomy. These provide an ideal aid for tooth anatomy and carving exercise.

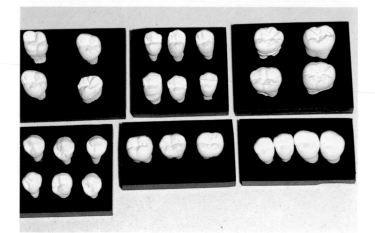

Fig 222 Various arrangements of stone samples.

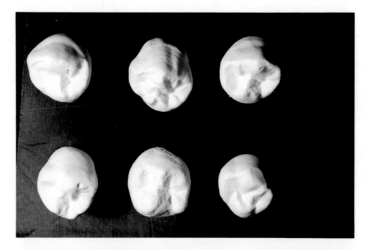

Fig 223 Stone sample of first and second mandibular bicuspids.

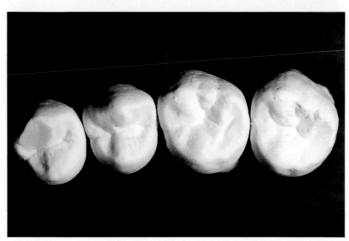

Fig 224 Stone sample of maxillary quadrant.

Duplication of natural teeth into dental stone often aids the visualizing of anatomy in particular occlusal characteristics. This is because dental stone is opaque and contours can be viewed in shadow.

The lack of a basic understanding of the character of natural dentition will severely impair any technical endeavour.

Once accuracy and understanding of tooth anatomy is acquired, improvements in contouring will occur; however, constraints are often present due to preparation design and available room as well as consideration for aesthetics and occlusion. It is by developing technical skills and the recognition of many different anatomic forms that problems are overcome.

7.7 Terminology and Uses for Specialized Ceramic Blends

Confusion is often caused through the use of inaccurate terminology. As an example, for many years enamel porcelain has been incorrectly described as either tip or incisal colour porcelain. Current thinking in the art of ceramics is to build dentine, secondary dentine and enamel with a similar structural form to natural dentition. This is a departure from the traditional method of body and tip building. It follows, therefore, that the term incisal porcelain is no longer applicable and that we are applying an 'enamel layer'.

Advances have been achieved with the formulation of many ceramic blends developed to simulate such natural characteristics as opacious dentine, high chroma dentines, root effects, secondary dentine and mamelon colours. These are the main areas of development, although other blends with the intention of matching specific areas of natural tooth structure can be found.

Opacious dentine*

Prepared blends of opacified dentines are designed for use beneath the dentine layer to reduce light transmission or mask opaque layers, and to create opaque dentine effects, opacious dentines are used in similar fashion to high chroma dentines, but need to be covered by a layer of dentine and have a different spectral effect.

High chroma dentines* (Korson, 1985)

Special blends of ceramic which match the colour of dentine and other intense dentine characteristics, that is, cervical and root colours, not to be confused with opacious dentine or secondary dentine blends.

High chroma dentines are used aproximally and also to create greater depth in the occlusal table to allow dentine colour to filter through the fissue pattern, in the palatal fossae and to simulate exposed root formation.

Secondary dentines (Creative Color System)

These are similar to high chroma dentines but have increased density and contain greater opacity, they are useful for areas of attrition where exposed dentine has become stained by oral bacteria. The incisal edge of lower incisors and worn occlusal cusps on posterior teeth may be simulated with secondary dentines.

---

* Opacious dentines, first developed by Vita Zahnfabrik, D-7880 Bad Sackingen, Postfach 1338, Germany.

* Developed by David Korson and first produced by Davis Schottlander & Davis, Letchworth, Herts. England.

Mamelon blends

These specialized blends are matched specifically to dentine mamelons and are invaluable for precisely matching this characteristic.

Opalescent frits

Much of the work on opalescence in dental porcelain originates from the work of Abbey (1962). Recent developments for custom built ceramics were brought to the fore by Makoto Yamamoto (1989) and developed with Shofu Vintage Porcelain.

Opalescent porcelains are now available from ceramic manufacturers including Ivoclar Classic, Vita Omega and Ducera LFC Opal. These frits have natural opalescence and provide a useful enamel effect (see page 108).

References

1. *Abbey A:* Improvements In and Relating To Ceramic Artificial Teeth and a Process for the Preparation Thereof. British Patent No 897.686. 1962.
2. *Geller W:* Davis Schottlander and Davis. Seminar. London 1990.
3. *Korson D. L:* The Simulation of Natural Tooth Colours in the Ceramo-metal System with Highly Chromatized Dentine Powders. Quintessence of Dental Technology. Quintessence Publishing Co. July/August 1985.
4. *McLean J. W:* Science and Art of Dental Ceramics Vol II pp 290-291. Quintessence Publishing Co. 1980.
5. *Toogood G. D. & Archibald J. R:* Technique for Establishing Porcelain Margins. Journal of Prosthetic Dentistry. 40:464 1978.
6. *Vryonis P:* A Simplified Approach to the Complete Porcelain Margin. J. Prosthet. Dent. 42(5): 592-593 1979.
7. *Vryonis P:* A Manual for the Fabrication of the Complete Porcelain Margin. Melbourne, 3000 Victoria. Australia. Published by the author.
8. *Yamamoto M:* Metal Ceramics. pp285-289 Quintessence Pub Co Inc. Chicago. 1985.
9. *Yamamoto M:* A newly developed "opal" ceramic and its clinical use, with special attention to its relative refractive index. QDT Yearbook. Quintessence Pub Co. 1989.

8 Case Studies

Two in depth case studies are featured to illustrate the practical results achieved. In addition, a number of completed cases are presented.

8.1 Anterior Splinted Crowns

Laboratory Technique to Develop Wax Trials Through to the Definitive Metal/ Ceramic Restoration

The detailed case is a periodontal splint involving six maxillary anterior splinted crowns.

The established aesthetic anatomy accomplished through wax trials has to be transferred accurately to the ceramic restoration. This will involve techniques to control the position of both metal substrate design and porcelain build-up.

As with many patients who require multiple anterior restorative treatment, interdental spacing can be a problem. Special attention was given to this aspect when fabricating the wax trial. The contact between teeth should be kept long and with a gentle curvature into the marginal ridge (fig 225).

Silicone* indices are fabricated to record the position of the wax trial (figs 227 to 231).

As this case is a periodontal splint, supra-gingival margins have been prepared. (Becker et al, 1981 and Kramer, 1980) Metal collars are designed with a flat profile, in harmony with the emerging physiological contour.

Adequate space is allowed for interproximal contouring during the planning stages of the wax design for the metal substrate. This is an area where insufficient space can cause problems in creating realistic separation between teeth and the development of natural marginal contours (figs 232 to 234).

* Zetalabor silicone. Zhermack, 45021 Badia Polesine (Rovigo), Italy.

133

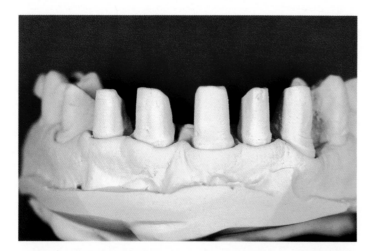

Fig 225 Study cast of the preparation, note the supra-gingival margins.

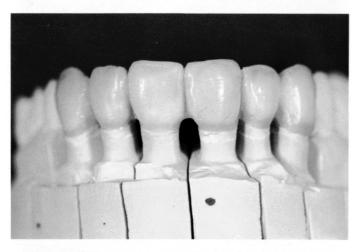

Fig 226 Wax trial on the working cast.

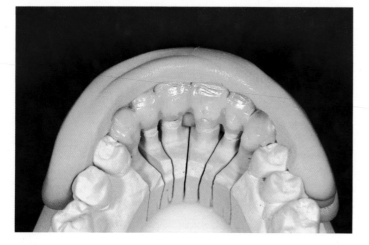

Fig 227 Facial contours and incisal edge position are recorded with a laboratory silicone matrix. The wax trial is retained, whilst the silicone matrix is used as a guide during waxing of the substrate.

Figs 228 and 229 The labial matrix is sectioned through the centre of each central incisor. This is necessary to facilitate a cross-section view.

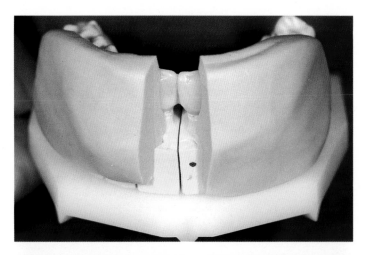

Fig 228

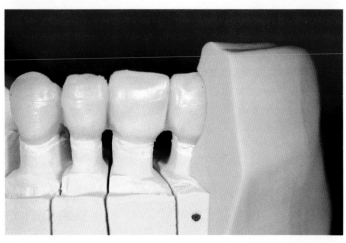

Fig 229

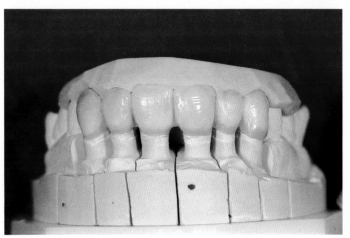

Fig 230 The incisal matrix is taken and trimmed level with the facial edges of the wax teeth.

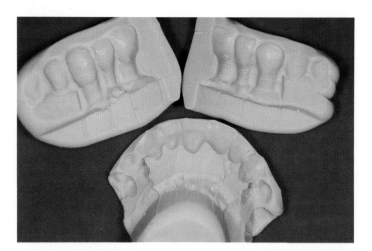

Fig 231 The three silicone matrices.

Figs 232 to 234 Wax substrate design.

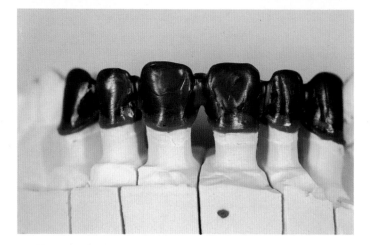

Figs 232 and 234 Facial and incisal aspects, note the shape and position of the proximal joins which are positioned in the palatal aspect, providing ample room for interdental shaping of the ceramic. In addition, the morphologic contour of each tooth.

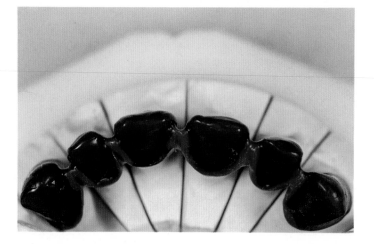

Fig 233 Palatal aspect depicts the high struts required for strength, this design is necessary due to the palatal placement of the proximal connectors.

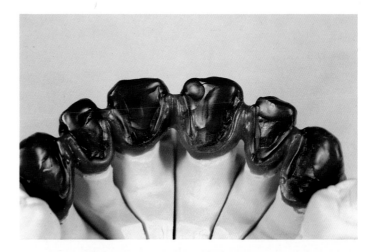

Fig 234

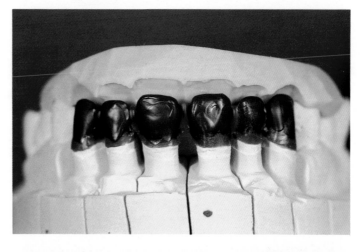

Figs 235 to 237 Wax substrate is checked in relation to the silicone matrices.

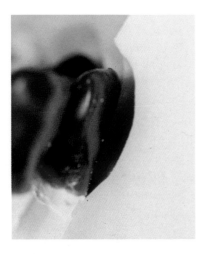

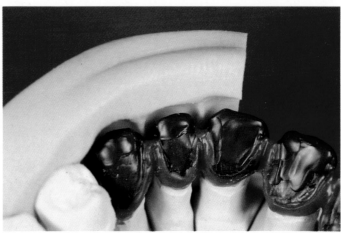

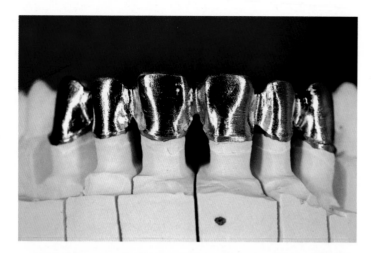

Figs 238 and 239 Trimmed metal substrates ready for oxide firing and porcelain application.

Fig 238

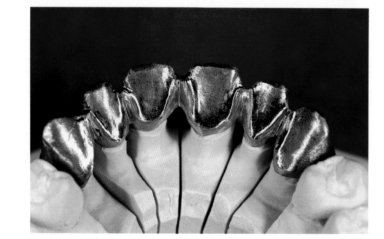

Fig 239

Porcelain Application

To achieve a depth of colour, High Chroma Dentine (HCD) (Korson, 1990) is laid between the teeth and also at the cervical of the central and canine teeth. By varying the amount of HCD in this region lighter or darker shades are achieved. In this case the layering for the canine extends into the mid-body section of the tooth, whilst in the central it was confined to the cervical third. The lateral was left entirely without HCD (fig 240).

Porcelain is only built to the labial aspect at this stage, utilizing the incisal index to ensure correct labial inclination, height and incisal edge position (fig 241. (Martignoni and Schonenberger, 1990)

The labial indices are not used during the build-up stages, as they inhibit the application of porcelain layers (fig 242). Cut back and incisal

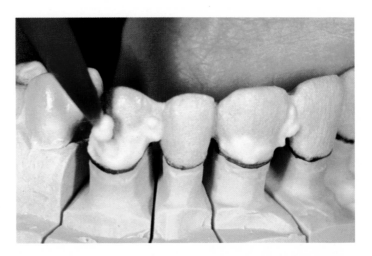

Fig 240 High chroma dentine is placed in the aproximal, cervical and body regions.

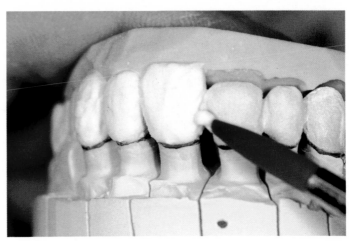

Fig 241 Dentine build-up, using the silicone matrix to establish the correct position of incisal edge position and facial inclination.

characterisation are carried out, followed by the building of enamel layers.

Several firings may be necessary to achieve the desired anatomy and at this stage the silicone indices are used as a guide to position. However, slavish grinding of porcelain to fully seat the silicone indices is counterproductive and will lead to a loss of artistry.

Following grinding adjustments in which occlusion and anatomy have been developed, green occlusal spray is used to aid visualization of the aesthetic contour and surface texture. Further refinements are carried out, followed by the smoothing of grinding marks and rough areas with a grey silicone wheel.*

The restoration is tried in and after adjustments, glazed and polished.

* Exa Intrapol Polisher. Edenta AG Ch-9434 AN/SG Hauptstrasse 7, St Gallen, Switzerland.

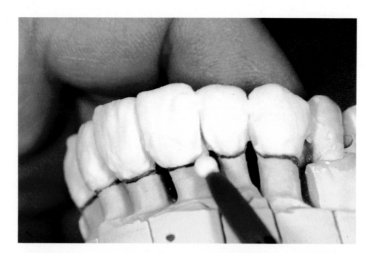

Fig 242 Labial veneer is completed.

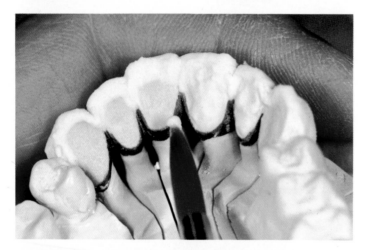

Fig 243 Palatal aspect is developed only after all aspects of layering and characterisation on the facial aspect are complete.

Incisal opaque can be seen as a guide to the placement of the labial veneer. High chroma dentine is placed in position.

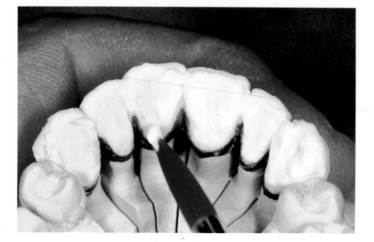

Fig 244 The marginal ridges and cingulum are developed in opalescent porcelain (white enamel).

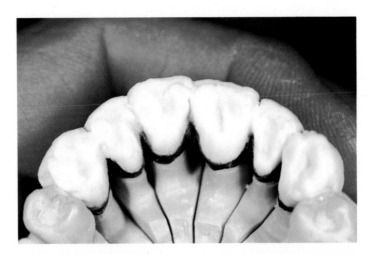

Fig 245 Complete palatal build-up.

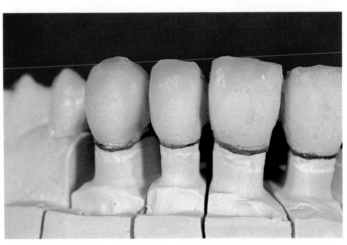

Fig 246 Situation after first firing.

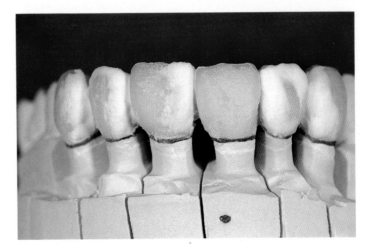

Figs 247 and 248 Porcelain addition to complete anatomy.

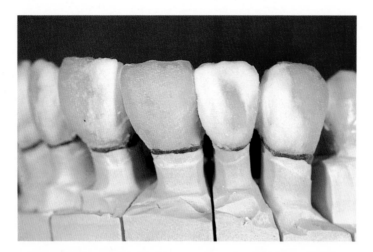

Fig 248

Figs 249 to 252 Refining the contours.

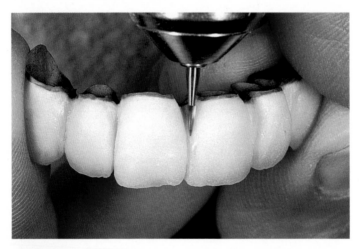

Fig 249 The non-edge technique developed by M. Yamamoto is useful in interproximal zones, where it may be difficult to use other instruments.

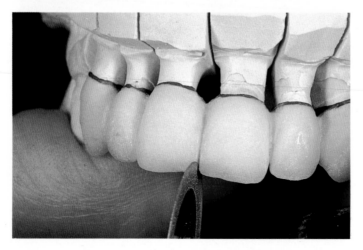

Fig 250 A fine flexible diamond disc is used for refinement of the interproximal region.

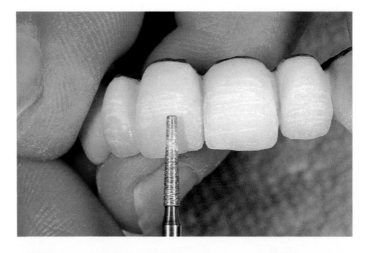

Fig 251 Surface detail is developed with a medium grit tapered diamond.

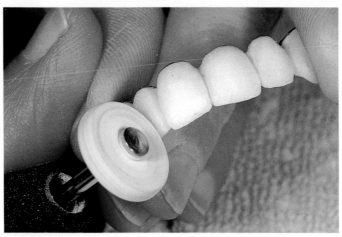

Fig 252 A silicone rubber wheel is employed to smooth high spots, such as the developmental lobes and other areas which become smooth through natural wear.

Figs 253 and 254 Green articulating spray is used to provide a clear idea of surface texture.

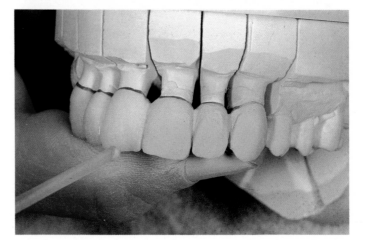

Fig 253

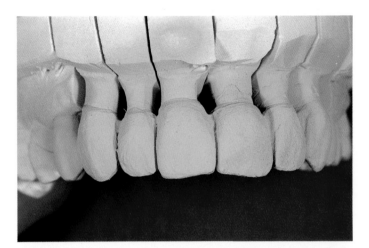

Fig 254

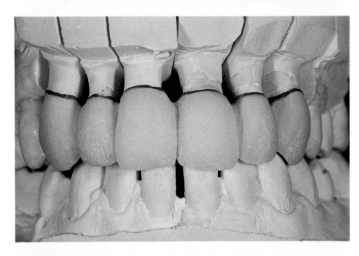

Fig 255 Bisque stage ready for try-in with the patient.

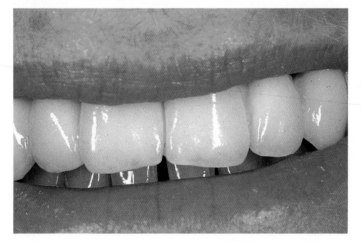

Fig 256 Final result. Salient points which bring a natural vitality to the ceramic are:

Close attention to anatomy through the use of wax trials.
Interproximal chroma using high chroma dentines.
Natural surface texture and lustre (dentist, W. Staden).

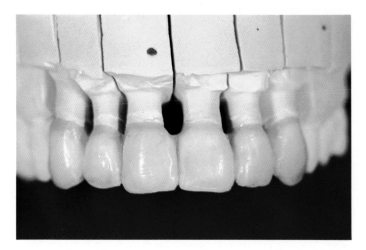

Fig 257 Wax trial for comparison with final result.

8.2 Restoration of the Mandibular Right Central and Lateral Incisors

Laboratory Technique to Develop Wax Trials through to the Definitive Empress* Restoration

The patient presented with poorly aligned mandibular central and lateral incisors, requesting that these be straightened to achieve a more aesthetic appearance.

The remaining tooth tissue was vital and, therefore, a pleasing colour; occlusal forces were not considered to be excessive. For these reasons it was decided to fabricate Empress crowns.

*Ivoclar, Schaan, Liechtenstein.

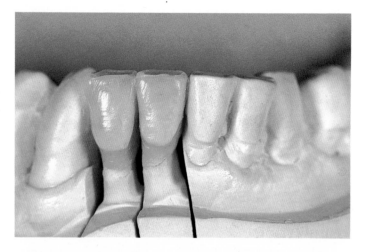

Figs 258 and 259 Wax trials after try-in and corrections are retained for future reference.

Fig 258

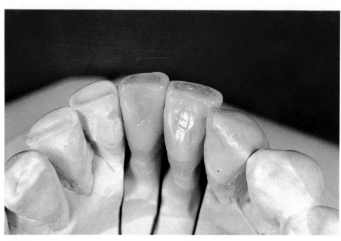

Fig 259

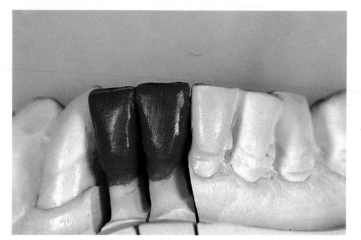

Fig 260 Wax crowns prior to spruing and investing for the Empress technique.

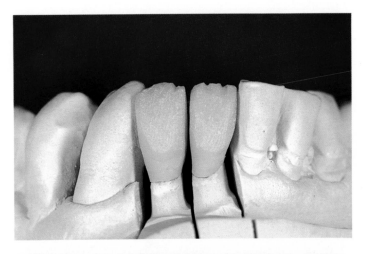

Fig 261 Pressed Empress crowns (layer technique) after adjustments to the dentine core.

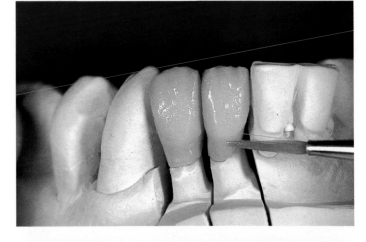

Fig 262 Preparation of the pressed cores for bonding of the enamel layers. Neutral powder is mixed with stain fluid, at the same time colour characteristics are applied with surface stains.

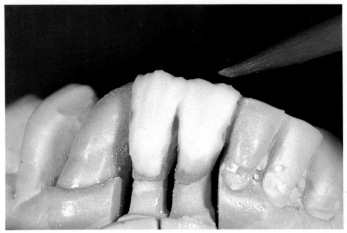

Fig 263 Enamel layers are built with reference to the wax trials.

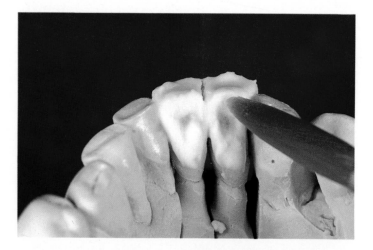

Fig 264 Neutral powder and stains are mixed with Color Clue Liquid to achieve the correct colour, and inlaid into the incisal edge wear facet.

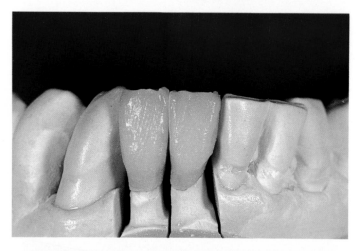

Fig 265 Crowns after sintering.

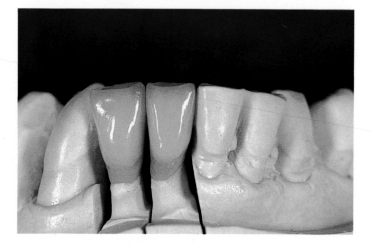

Fig 266 Glazed and polished crowns seen here on the working cast.

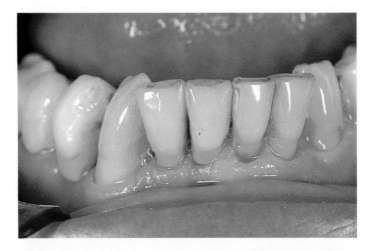

Figs 267 to 269 Completed case.

Fig 268 and 269 A key element in the success of this case is the careful control of surface lustre.

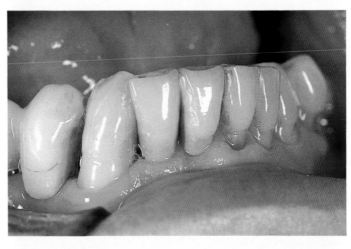

Fig 268

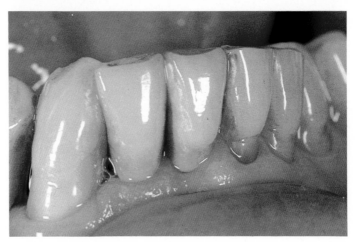

Fig 269 Close detail.

8.3 Restoration of a Lateral Incisor

The patient presented with an existing full porcelain crown which was unacceptable.

The obvious aesthetic faults were:

1. Poor anatomical shape.
2. Incorrect shade.
3. Soft tissue reacting unfavourably to the crown.

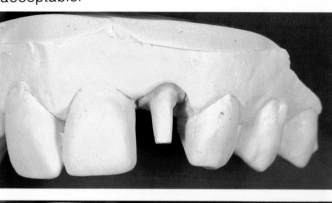

Fig 270a Cast of preparation for the Empress crown.

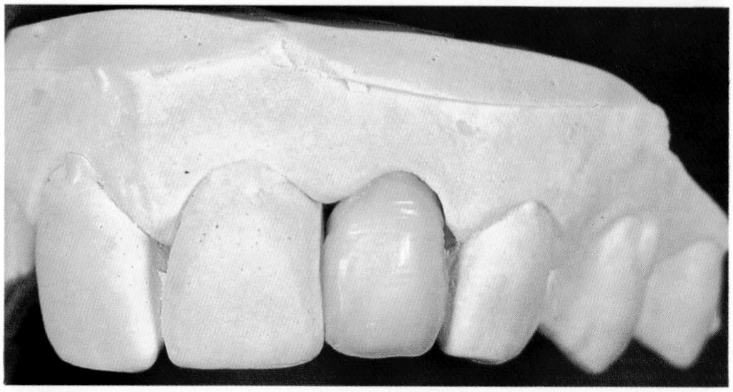

Fig 270b Wax trial. The most important aspect is the addition of wax to build out the mesial cervical corner.

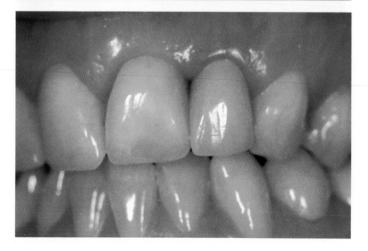

Fig 271 Patient's previous crown demonstrates the poor aesthetic consequences when anatomy and colour are neglected.

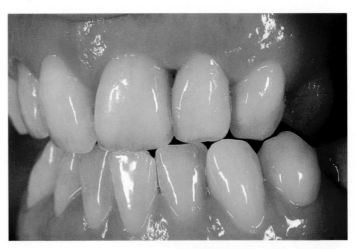

Fig 272 Empress crown. Lateral incisor.

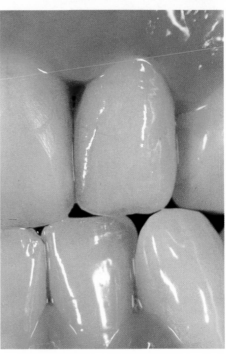

Fig 273 Close detail.

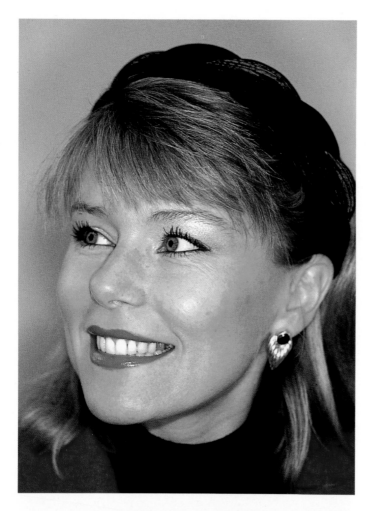

8.4 Restoration of Lateral and Canine Incisors

An attractive patient is unhappy with the poor aesthetics of her existing porcelain crowns. She feels very self-conscious and is afraid to smile, consequently this is affecting her confidence.

Figs 274 and 275 Previous unsightly metal-ceramic restorations mar an attractive smile.

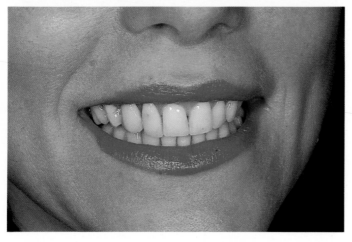

Fig 275

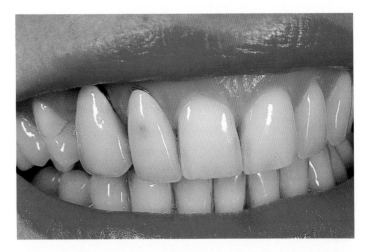

Fig 276 Close detail of previous unattractive restoration.

Figs 277 and 278 Completed metal-ceramic restoration.

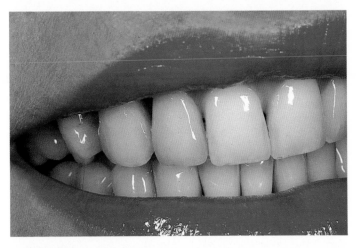

Fig 277

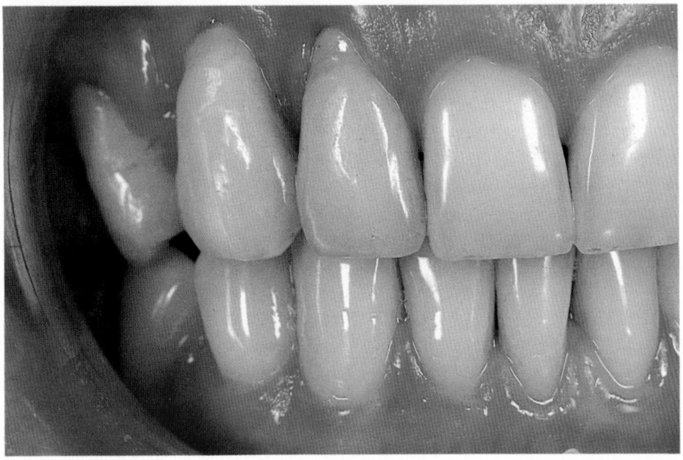

Fig 278

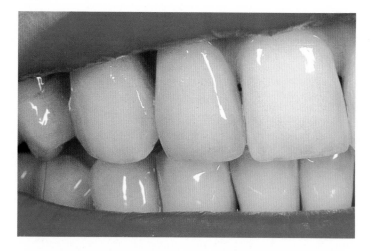

Fig 279 Close detail (dentist, W. Staden).

8.5 Case Presentations

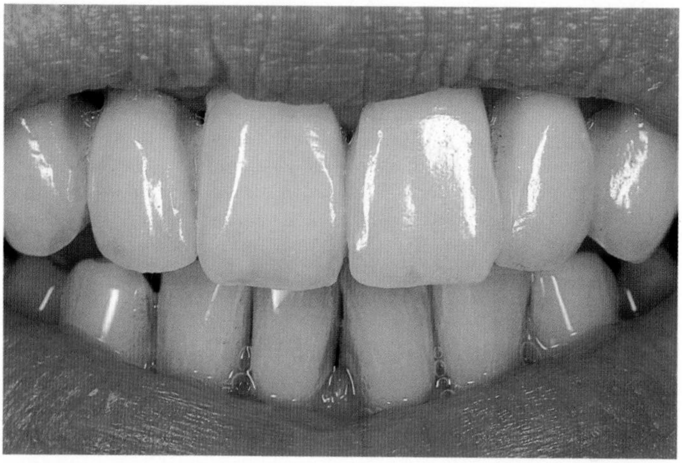

Figs 280 to 281b Bridge restoration of six anterior teeth to replace missing central incisors with a metal-ceramic bridge.

Fig 280

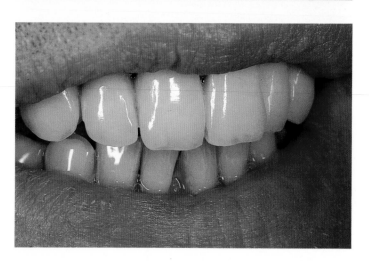

Fig 281a

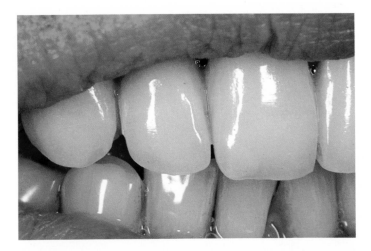

Fig 281b   Close detail.

Figs 282 and 283   Restoration of the left central incisor. Porcelain crown. All the effects have been built within the ceramic. The small discoloured spot was not included by request of the patient.

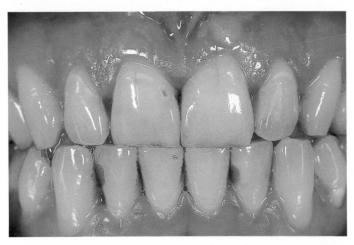

Fig 282

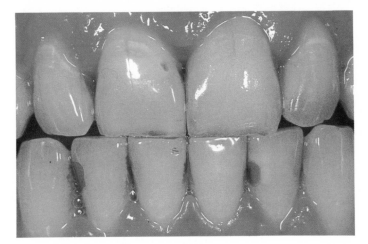

Fig 283

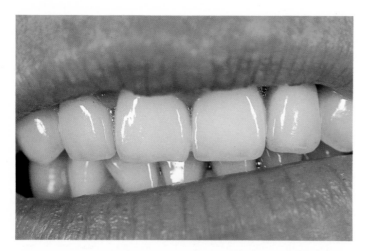

Fig 284   Metal-ceramic maxillary splint, involving six anterior teeth. The patient requested a light colour and an even arrangement.

Figs 285 and 286   Maxillary restoration of the anterior teeth with metal-ceramic crowns.

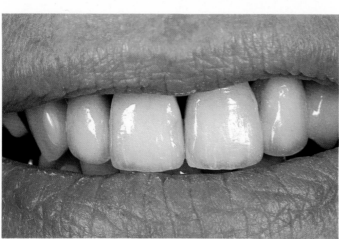

Fig 285

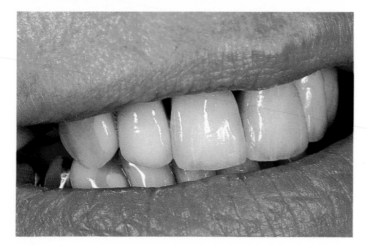

Fig 286

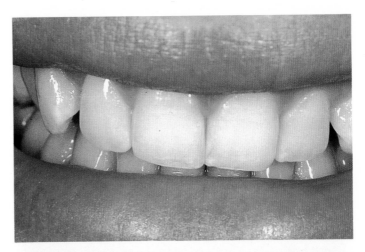

Fig 287 Maxillary left lateral and right central and lateral incisors restored with Empress crowns.

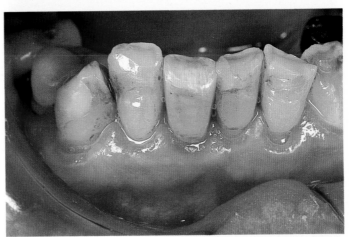

Fig 288 Mandibular incisor restored with a full porcelain crown.

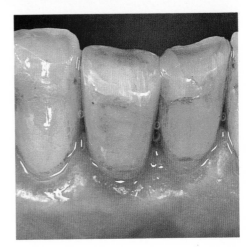

Fig 289 Close detail.

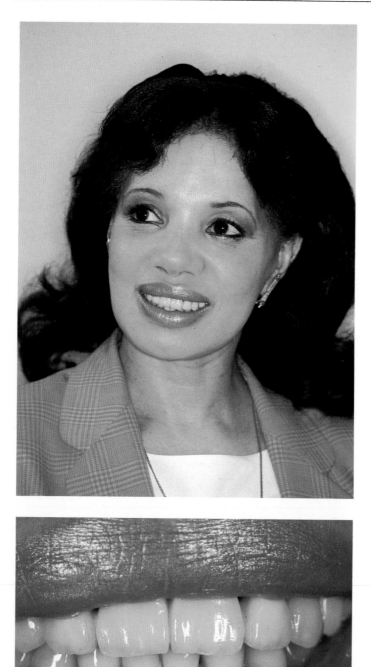

Fig 290 to 292. Part of a full maxillary reconstruction. Six anterior metal-ceramic splinted crowns. (Ivoclar Classic V).

Fig 290

Fig 291

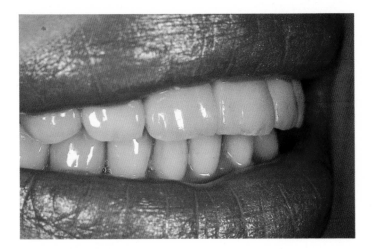

Fig 292 Lateral view.

References

1. *Becker C. M. et al:* Crown Contours that promote access for oral hygiene. Quintessence Int. February 1981: 12(2): 233.
2. *Korson D. L:* Natural Ceramics. Quintessence Pub. Co. London. England 1990.
3. *Kramer G. M:* Rationale of Periodontal Therapy. Reportato de Goldman and Cohen in Periodontal Therapy. CV Mosby Co. St Louis. 1980 6 Ed.
4. *Martignoni M.* & *Schönenberger A:* Precision Fixed Prosthodontics. Clinical and Laboratory Aspects. Quintessence Pub. Co. Chicago, Illinois 1990 pp240-241.
5. Yamamoto M: Fundamentals of Esthetics. QDT 1990/91 pp70-71.